EMQs For MRCOG Part 2 in Obstetrics

Authors

Prabha Sinha
FRCOG, MRCPI, Dip Med Ed, Dip Mgmt
Consultant Obstetrician and Gynaecologist
East Sussex Hospitals NHS Trust

M. Mishra
MS, MRCOG

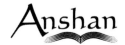

EMQs FOR MRCOG PART 2 IN OBSTETRICS

Published by:
Anshan Ltd
11a Little Mount Sion
Tunbridge Wells
Kent. TN1 1YS

Tel: +44 (0) 1892 557767
Fax: +44 (0) 1892 530358

e-mail: info@anshan.co.uk
website: www.anshan.co.uk

ISBN: 978 1 848290 617

British Library Cataloguing in Publication Data

A catalogue record for this book is available from the British Library.

Copy Editor: Catherine Lain
Cover Design: Terry Griffith
Cover Image: Shutterstock
Typeset by: GCS, Leighton Buzzard, Beds.
Printed and bound by: CPI Antony Rowe, Chippenham, Wiltshire

Contents

Preface

The Royal College of Obstetricians and Gynaecologists (RCOG) introduced Extended Matching Questions (EMQs) some time ago, partially replacing the old-style MCQs and short essays. As EMQs provide greater consistency and fairness, are more transparent and test the depth of knowledge of the candidates in the exam, more emphasis has been put on them.

Generally EMQs are very similar to multiple choice questions. However, the main difference is that EMQs test the depth of applied knowledge, making the exams more authentic, transparent and valid. The probability of getting the correct answer by chance is very low and therefore candidates must have an adequate knowledge prior to attempting the questions.

From March 2011 the format of the Part 2 MRCOG written examination has changed and the number of EMQs has increased from 40 to 90. EMQs now make up 40% of overall marks whereas before they only accounted for 15%. There are three papers in the written examination. The number of questions and the time allotted to answer them have been changed accordingly.

The distribution of the marks is as follows (RCOG website):

	Proportion of Overall Marks
Paper 1 (4 SAQs) – 105 minutes	30%
Paper 2 (120 MCQs, 45 EMQs – 135 minutes)	30%
Paper 3 (120 MCQs, 45 EMQs) – 135 minutes	40%

As this book contains evidence-based answers, candidates will find them easy to follow. The book features 160 questions covering most of the subject of obstetrics practice and is primarily based on guidelines published by the RCOG, the National Institute for Health and Clinical Excellence (NICE) and the most up-to-date research and consensus.

All the questions are based on real clinical scenario commonly encountered in day-to-day clinical practice such as that from outpatient clinics, acute admissions from accident and emergency and labour wards.

It is essential to practice EMQs before taking the exam. However, basic detailed knowledge is necessary and studying textbooks is required to gain knowledge in preparation for the exam. Books such as those containing short essays, MCQs and EMQs are not a replacement for textbooks. This book will coach students to answer EMQs effectively once they have acquired a basic knowledge. Revision of the guidelines should ensue.

Full details about the exam itself are available on the RCOG website. This book follows the established format; just choose the most appropriate answer for each question. It is important to read the statements carefully to identify the theme and then select the most relevant and appropriate answer.

For the revision of the Part 2 MRCOG exam this book is essential.

Syllabus

The syllabus is freely available on the RCOG website. It is comprised of almost 18 modules and includes basic clinical and surgical skills, audit, research, clinical risk (clinical governance), teaching and appraisal.

In obstetrics the syllabus covers early pregnancy, antenatal, intrapartum and postnatal care, maternal and fetal medicine. In gynaecology the main modules include detailed knowledge regarding common gynaecological diseases, infertility/ subfertility, contraception and sexual health, pelvic floor including urological problems, oncology and perioperative and post-operative care.

These modules are based on standard textbooks and guidelines, teaching material provided by the RCOG e.g. *TOG*, StratOG, DIALOG.

Examination preparation not only includes detailed subject knowledge but also that of recent evidence related to the subject, published in the Green-top guidelines by RCOG, NICE and other relevant places (CEMACH, National Screening).

Journals such as *BJOG* and *TOG* are also relevant as they too discuss recent development.

Abbreviations

A&E	Accident and Emergency
AC	Abdominal Circumference
ALT	Alanine Transaminase
ANC	Antenatal care
APTT	Activated partial thomboplastin time
ASS	Acute splenic sequestration
BMI	Body mass index
BP	Blood pressure
BPD	Biparietal diameter
CS	Caesarean section
CT	Computed tomographic
CTG	Cardiotocographic
CTPA	Computed Tomographic Pulmonary Angiogram
CVS	Chorionic Villus Sampling
DIC	Disseminated intravascular coagulation
DVT	Deep venous thrombosis
EAS	External anal sphincter
ECV	External cephalic version
EFW	Effective fetal weight
FBS	Fetal blood sampling
FFP	Fresh frozen plasma
FGM	Female genital mutilation
GDM	Gestational diabetes mellitus
GP	General Practitioner
HAART	Highly Active Anti-Retroviral Therapy
HbS	Sickle cell haemoglobin
HELLP	Haemolytic anaemia, elevated liver enzyme, low platelet
HIV	Human immunodeficiency virus
HSV	Herpes simplex virus
IAS	Internal anal sphincter
ICU	Intensive care unit
IM	Intramuscular
IUGR	Intrauterine Growth Restriction
IUFD	Intrauterine fetal death

IV	Intravenous
IVF	In-vitro fertilization
KFT	Kidney function test
LFT	Liver function tests
LMWH	Low molecular weight heparin
LSCS	Lower section caesarean section
MCA	Middle cerebral artery
MMR	Measles, Mumps and Rubella
MRI	Magnetic resonance imaging
NT	Nuchal translucency
OGTT	Oral glucose tolerance test
OHSS	Ovarian hyperstimulation syndrome
PAPP	Pregnancy-associated plasma protein
PE	Pulmonary Embolism
PIH	Pregnancy-induced hypertension
PPH	Postpartum haemorrhage
PPROM	Preterm premature rupture of membrane
PTE	Pulmonary thromboembolism
RCT	Randomised control trial
RDS	Respiratory distress syndrome
rHuEPO	Recombinant human erythropoietin
SCBU	Special care baby unit
SGA	Small for gestational age
SROM	Spontaneous rupture of membrane
TTTS	Twin to twin transfusion syndrome
TVS	Transvaginal scan
UDCA	Ursodeoxycholic acid
USG	Ultrasound
VBAC	Vaginal birth after caesarean section
VTE	Venous thromboembolism
VZV	Varicella zoster virus
VZIG	Varicella zoster immune globulin
ZDV	Zidouvidine

About the authors

Prabha Sinha is a Consultant Obstetrician and Gynaecologist at the Conquest Hospital in St Leonards-on-Sea, East Sussex, UK. She is also Honorary Consultant in Fetal Medicine at Guy's and St. Thomas' Hospitals in London. She has Fellowship of the Royal College of Obstetricians and Gynaecologists (FRCOG) and Membership of the Royal College of Physicians of Ireland (MRCPI). She is involved with undergraduate students from Brighton and GKT Medical School, as well as postgraduate education and assessment. She is currently an examiner for the Membership of the Royal College of Obstetricians and Gynaecologists (MRCOG), as well as the GMC exam for overseas doctors. She has also been a teacher on MRCOG courses locally, nationally, at the RCOG and internationally.

She has published many articles in peer reviewed journals and made a huge number of presentations and lectures in various national and international conferences.

She has written EMQ books for MRCOG Part 1, 2, DRCOG and OSCE for Colposcopy.

This is her eighth authored book.

Mamta Mishra is a member of Royal College of Obstetricians and Gynaecologists (MRCOG) with ten years of experience in obstetrics and gynaecology. She has a great interest in teaching and training and participates in organizing and running MRCOG Part 1 and 2 courses twice a year in New Delhi.

EMQs on Anaemia, Blood Transfusion and Anti-D

Options for questions 1 – 3

A	Recombinant human erythropoietin (rHuEPO)	H	Recombinant factor VIIa
B	Parenteral iron	I	Cell salvage
C	Tranexamic acid and recombinant factor VIIa	J	Blood transfusion in conjunction with haematologist
D	Blood transfusion	K	Autologous transfusion
E	Mefenamic acid	L	Fresh frozen plasma
F	Platelet transfusion only	M	Oral calcium and oral iron
G	Oral iron	N	Vitamin B12 and iron

Instruction: For each question posed below, choose the single most appropriate management from the list above. The given option may be used once, more than once or not at all.

Question 1	A 30 year old is booked at 24 weeks in her fourth pregnancy. Her haemoglobin level is 9 g/dl. She has had the blood test and screening done for haemoglobinopathies that did not show any abnormalities. Blood film showed microcytic hypochromic anaemia.
Answer 1	
Question 2	An 18 year old African woman in her first pregnancy is booked at 10 weeks. She is feeling tired, lethargic and breathless. On investigation, her haemoglobin level is found to be 7 g/dl. Hb electrophoresis done confirmed sickle cell anaemia.
Answer 2	
Question 3	A 32 year old primigravida has had spontaneous vaginal delivery of a male baby weighing 3.5kg. Soon after delivery of the placenta, she started bleeding profusely. Corrective measures such as replacement of plasma coagulation factors, fibrinogen and platelet have failed to control bleeding effectively.
Answer 3	

Answers and explanations

Answer 1 (G) Oral iron

Iron deficiency anaemia in the antenatal period is defined as a haemoglobin (Hb) level less than 10.5 g/dl. Haemoglobinopathies should be excluded before the diagnosis of iron deficiency anaemia is made, especially in primigravida.

According to the National Institute for Health and Clinical Excellence (NICE) anaemia is defined as an Hb level of <11.0 g/dL and <10.5 g/dL at booking and 28 weeks respectively.

Iron deficiency accounts for 85% of all cases of anaemia. Low iron stores or nutritional deficiency results from previous successive pregnancies or previous heavy menstrual blood loss. It is characterised by low mean cell volume and mean cell haemoglobin concentration.

The normal physiological change of an increase in plasma volume causes haemodilution during pregnancy. Although the red cell mass increases, plasma volume increases disproportionately, resulting in a lowering of the Hb to approximately 11.5 g/dL.

Other causes of anemia are:

- folic acid deficiency
- sickle cell disease
- haemoglobin SC
- beta thalassaemia (more common in patients from South East Asia, Southern Europe and Africa)
- vitamin B12 deficiency
- chronic haemolysis (hereditary spherocytosis)
- paroxysmal nocturnal haemoglobinuria
- leukaemia
- gastrointestinal bleeding.

Oral or parenteral iron therapy is commonly prescribed to correct the deficiency depending on the gestational age and the compliance.

Oral iron should be the preferred first-line treatment for iron deficiency before 36 weeks' gestation (200mg elemental iron per day). It is usually adequate, well tolerated and a cost-effective way to replace iron stores in most patients.

Recent research shows oral iron plus folate to be more effective than iron alone, irrespective of serum folate levels. Blood transfusion should be avoided as much as possible.

The indications for the administration of intravenous iron are:

- patients with persistent anaemia, who claim to have been on oral iron for some time
- not well tolerated causing gastrointestinal side effects (constipation or diarrhoea, nausea)
- poor compliance and inadequate absorption.

Administration of oral iron takes 2–2·5 weeks for the Hb to start rising and the normal level is reached in approximately 8 weeks. It takes 6 months for iron stores to be repleted. With intravenous iron, Hb starts rising in 1 week and the percentage of responders is higher.

Answer 2 (J) Blood transfusion in conjunction with haematologist

Other types of anaemia (bone marrow failure and haemoglobinopathies syndromes), should be managed by blood transfusion. Proper consultation and discussion with a haematologist is necessary where appropriate.

In sickle cell disease transfusions are not required for anaemia or during episodes of pain in non-pregnant women. However, urgent replacement of blood is often required for sudden severe anaemia due to ASS, parvovirus B19 infection, or in hyperhaemolytic crises during pregnancy and can be administered as top-up or as exchange transfusions.

Exchange transfusion decreases the concentration of HbS, therefore it is preferable to a top-up when the patient is unwell. This increases the overall oxygen-carrying capacity of the blood.

Prophylactic transfusion should be used on an individual basis depending on the physician's experience, the type of facilities available, the severity of the sickle cell disease and obstetric factors (e.g. twins).

Answer 3 (H) Recombinant factor VIIa

Severe postpartum haemorrhage remains an important cause of maternal morbidity and mortality. The most common cause of postpartum hemorrhage is uterine atony. For first-line management of postpartum haemorrhage adequate blood and fluid replacement is mandatory. Further therapeutic measures consist of a variety of medical interventions and surgical techniques.

Administrations of uterotonics (and more recently recombinant activated factor VII) are most commonly used and provide effective medical therapy in controlling postpartum haemorrhage.

There is conflicting evidence regarding the use of fibrinolytic agents (such as tranexamic acid) and there is no evidence to suggest its role in obstetric haemorrhage.

Options for questions 4 – 6

A	No anti-D prophylaxis	F	Blood transfusion
B	FFP of different ABO group is acceptable. No anti-D prophylaxis is required	G	FFP of different ABO group is acceptable. Anti-D prophylaxis is required
C	Anti-Rh D immunoglobulin (at a dose of 250 IU)	H	Platelet transfusion along with anti-D prophylaxis is required
D	Platelet transfusion is recommended	I	Anti-D prophylaxis is required
E	Platelet along with cryoprecipitate to be transfused	J	Platelet transfusion without anti-D prophylaxis is required

Instruction: For each question posed below, choose the single most appropriate management from the A–J list above. The given option may be used once, more than once or not at all.

Question 4	A 36 year old multigravida has had spontaneous vaginal delivery of a female baby, weighing 4.5kg. She started bleeding actively soon after birth. On investigation, her platelet count is 40 x 10^9/l and blood group is B negative. Rh D-negative platelet is not available.
Answer 4	
Question 5	A 40 year old conceived with IVF pregnancy. She had spontaneous vaginal delivery of a female infant weighing 3.5kg. Immediately afterwards, she started bleeding profusely. Her platelet count is 40 x 10^9/l and blood group is B negative. Caesarean hysterectomy has been performed to stop bleeding after all measures had failed.
Answer 5	
Question 6	A 30 year old primigravida has had a vaginal delivery at 34 weeks. She had severe pregnancy-induced hypertension with proteinuria and felt unwell. She delivered very quickly followed by brisk loss. She started to ooze from the cannula site soon after delivery. Her blood group is A negative. A haematologist has been contacted for an appropriate management.
Answer 6	

Answers and explanations

Answer 4 (H) Platelet transfusion along with anti-D prophylaxis is required

If a woman is actively bleeding then platelet count should be checked frequently to make sure the count does not fall below the 50 x 10^9/l, which provides a margin of safety. In an actively bleeding patient platelet transfusion should be considered if the level starts falling below the safe level of 75 x 10^9/l.

Rh D-negative women should receive Rh D-negative platelets and should be group compatible.

A dose of 250 IU of anti-Rh D immunoglobulin should be given if Rh D-positive platelet (if Rh D-negative platelet is not available) has been transfused in an Rh D-negative woman.

Answer 5 (J) Platelet transfusion without anti-D prophylaxis is required

Anti-Rh D immunoglobulin (at a dose of 250 IU) should be given if the platelets are Rh D-positive and the woman is Rh D-negative. However, if a caesarean hysterectomy has been performed anti-D is not necessary as further pregnancy is not anticipated.

Answer 6 (B) FFP of different ABO group is acceptable. No anti-D prophylaxis is required

A combination of FFP, platelets and cryoprecipitate is indicated in the woman who is bleeding with a diagnosis of disseminated intravascular coagulation (DIC). Anti-D prophylaxis is not required if an Rh D-negative woman receives Rh D-positive FFP or cryoprecipitate.

Options for questions 7 – 9

A	Anti-D Ig should be given as soon as possible	F	250 IU of anti-D Ig and test to detect FMH
B	Anti-D Ig should be given at six-weekly intervals	G	500 IU of anti-D Ig and test to detect FMH
C	No need for anti-D Ig	H	500 IU of anti-D Ig
D	Anti-D Ig IM preparation (2500 IU or 5000 IU)	I	250 IU of anti-D Ig
E	Exchange transfusion	J	Intravenous anti-D Ig

Instruction: For each question posed below, choose the single most appropriate management answer from the A–J list above. The given option may be used once, more than once or not at all.

Question 7	A 30 year old primigravida has been transfused three units of Rh positive blood inadvertently after a road traffic accident. She is 10 weeks pregnant. Her blood group is A negative.
Answer 7	
Question 8	A woman has delivered at 38 weeks by LSCS. Her blood group is B negative. Blood group of her baby is B positive. She has received antenatal prophylaxis. The midwife is enquiring about further prophylaxis.
Answer 8	
Question 9	A 34 year old has threatened miscarriage at 10 weeks. Her bleeding has stopped and USG showed a viable fetus. She is AB negative and has received anti-D prophylaxis in her last two pregnancies.
Answer 9	

Answers and explanations

Answer 7 (E) Exchange transfusion

If exchange transfusion is done immediately, the load of Rh D-positive RBC in the circulation will go down significantly. One-blood-volume exchange will achieve a 65–70% of reduction in Rh D-positive cells and two-volume exchange to 85–90%.

Answer 8 (G) 500 IU of anti-D Ig and test to detect FMH

Following delivery, a screening test must be done to look for large feto-maternal haemorrhage by a Kleihauer test. This will help in identifying a woman who needs additional Rh immunoglobulin.

Answer 9 (C) No need for anti-D Ig

If a woman has threatened miscarriage and USG suggests a viable fetus of less than 12 weeks of pregnancy, anti-D is not required if bleeding has ceased.

In uncomplicated miscarriage or mild painless vaginal bleeding, prophylactic anti-D immunoglobulin is not necessary because the risk of feto-maternal haemorrhage (FMH) is negligible. However, 250 IU prophylactic anti-D immunoglobulin should be given in cases of therapeutic termination of pregnancy, whether by surgical or medical methods.

(Reference – RCOG Green-top guidelines nos. 47, 22)

EMQs on Postpartum Haemorrhage

Options for questions 10 – 12

A	Oxytocin 5 IU by IM injection	G	Oxytocin high dose infusion
B	Oxytocin 5 IU by slow IV injection	H	Uterine artery embolisation
C	Misoprostol	I	Uterine artery ligation
D	Syntometrine intramuscular injection	J	Caesarean hysterectomy
E	Ergometrine intramuscular injection	K	Ergometrine intravenous injection
F	Oxytocin low dose infusion	L	Internal iliac artery ligation

Instruction: For each question posed below, choose the single **most appropriate prophylactic oxytocic for management of the third stage of labour** from the list above. The given option may be used once, more than once or not at all.

Question 10	A 30 year old woman in her second pregnancy has had normal spontaneous vaginal delivery. She has no risk factor for PPH. She has consented for active management of the third stage of labour.
Answer 10	
Question 11	A 32 year old woman has had an emergency caesarean section for undiagnosed breech. She has had a previous delivery complicated by postpartum haemorrhage. She is very keen to have a prophylactic measure taken for the management of the third stage of labour.
Answer 11	
Question 12	A 20 year old primigravida has delivered at home. She is happy for prophylactic management of the third stage of labour but scared of an injection and keen to have alternative medication if possible. She has heard about other alternatives from her friend who has needle phobia.
Answer 12	

Answers and explanations

Answer 10 (A) Oxytocin 5 IU by IM injection

Intramuscular injection of oxytocin (5 or 10 IU) is the drug of choice for prophylaxis in the third stage of labour during vaginal delivery without risk factors for PPH.

The third stage of labour is the period from the birth of the baby until delivery of the placenta. The degree of blood loss depends on how quickly the placenta separates from the uterine wall and myometrial contraction. Severe postpartum haemorrhage is a major problem and an important cause of maternal mortality in developing countries due to lack of access to treatment and anaemia.

Routine use of oxytocin may reduce the amount of blood loss during the third stage of labour, which has been supported by clinical trials. However, there is not enough evidence regarding its side effects to justify its routine use. More research is required in this area to weigh up the benefits of reduction in blood loss.

Answer 11 (B) Oxytocin 5 IU by slow IV injection

For women delivering by caesarean section, oxytocin (5 IU by slow intravenous injection) should be used to encourage myometrial contraction leading to reduction in blood loss. To enhance the uterine contraction IV is most appropriate as access is already there.

During CS, uterine incision and manual removal of the placenta (rather than waiting for spontaneous expulsion) often cause more bleeding than usual.

Answer 12 (C) Misoprostol

Misoprostol is associated with significant decreases in the rate of acute postpartum haemorrhage and mean blood loss. However, it is not as effective as oxytocin and side effects may be more in comparison. It may be used when the other agents such as syntocinon are not available or the patient does not like injections (or in a home-birth setting). Side effects are supposed to be less than syntometrin or ergometrine.

Misoprostol is cheap, administration is easy. Its stability and positive safety profile make it a good option in resource-poor settings.

Misoprostol can also be used for postpartum haemorrhage due to uterine atony in women who suffer from asthma.

Options for questions 13 – 14

A	A high concentration of oxygen (10–15 litres/minute)	F	Oxygen (10–15 litres/minute) and anaesthetic help
B	Urinary catheter	G	Send investigations
C	Two 14-gauge IV cannula	H	One 14-gauge IV cannula
D	Commence crystalloid infusion	I	Recombinant factor VIIa therapy
E	Keep the woman warm	J	Arrange blood

Instruction: For each question posed below, choose the single **most appropriate initial management** from the A–J list above. The given option may be used once, more than once or not at all.

Question 13	A 26 year old woman has delivered normally but had prolonged first stage of labour. Her BMI is 34. She has collapsed soon after delivery after severe PPH and bled approximately 1.5 litres.
Answer 13	

Question 14	A 32 year old woman delivered normally with a prolonged second stage of labour. She had an epidural and had normal vaginal delivery. She bled approximately 700ml soon after delivery and had no other risk factor for PPH.
Answer 14	

Answers and explanations

Answer 13 (F) Oxygen (10–15 litres/minute) and anaesthetic help

The patient should be resuscitated first followed by ABC (assess airway, breathing and evaluate circulation) and oxygen at 10–15 litres/minute by mask should be initiated as soon as possible.

Excessive bleeding or haemorrhage results in the loss of intravascular volume causing decreased oxygen delivery to tissues and organs. Initially tissue perfusion is maintained by reflex tachycardia, peripheral vasoconstriction, and increased myocardial contractility as physiological compensatory mechanisms.

Further reduction in blood volume results in circulatory collapse, end-organ damage and eventual death, therefore, immediate volume replacement is important.

Answer 14 (H) One 14-gauge IV cannula

In minor PPH (blood loss 500–1000ml) basic measures should be initiated in anticipation of a development in major haemorrhage. One 14-gauge cannula should be inserted for intravenous access if fluid replacement is required. Initially, crystalloids (0.9% normal saline, Ringer's lactate solution, compound electrolyte solution) administration is recommended.

As there are no signs of clinical shock in minor PPH these measures are prophylactic only. If blood loss becomes excessive then it should be treated as major PPH.

Options for questions 15 – 16

A	Haemostatic brace suturing	**F**	Bimanual uterine compression
B	Ergometrine 0.5mg	**G**	Syntocinon 5 units
C	Syntocinon infusion (40 units in 500 ml Hartmann's solution at 125 ml/hour)	**H**	Direct intramyometrial injection of carboprost 0.5mg
D	Ensure bladder is empty	**I**	Misoprostol 1000 micrograms rectally
E	Intrauterine balloon tamponade	**J**	Bilateral ligation of uterine arteries

Instruction: For each option posed below, choose the single **most appropriate initial management** from the A–J list above. The given option may be used once, more than once or not at all.

Question 15	A 30 year old multigravida woman delivered twins with a normal vaginal delivery. Soon after the third stage she started bleeding profusely. There is no perineal laceration and the uterus is very soft and not contracting properly.
Answer 15	
Question 16	A 32 year old woman in her first pregnancy has had normal vaginal delivery. Her second stage was prolonged. She had a small vaginal tear and required no suturing. Soon after delivery of the placenta, she started having profuse vaginal bleeding. Uterus was found to be relaxed and atonic. Pharmacological method and bimanual compression have failed to control bleeding. She wants to preserve her fertility.
Answer 16	

Answers and explanations

Answer 15 (F) Bimanual uterine compression

When uterine atony is a possible cause of the bleeding, bimanual uterine compression (rubbing up a contraction) to stimulate myometrium should be the first measure. Pharmacological measures should be considered in conjunction with the manual compression until the bleeding stops. Further measures are taken if required and after arrival of assistance.

During bimanual compression consistent pressure with two hands results in external compression of the uterus, which reduces blood flow. Simultaneously, the uterus is pushed anteriorly between two hands, putting the uterine arteries under tension. This further reduces blood flow to the uterus and thereby further blood loss. This is the quickest method of providing tamponade.

Answer 16 (E) Intrauterine balloon tamponade

If pharmacological measures fail to control the haemorrhage, surgical haemostasis should be attempted sooner rather than later.

Intrauterine balloon tamponade is an appropriate first-line 'surgical' intervention for most women where uterine atony is the only or main cause of haemorrhage.

A different variety of balloon or uterine packing is placed inside the uterus to provide direct compression of the uterine wall, decreasing the blood supply and further loss.

The method of uterine tamponade using balloons has recently been added to the armamentarium for managing PPH. There are various balloons available including the Bakri, Foley, Sengstaken-Blakemore, Rusch and condom catheter.

The balloon can be left in place for 8 to 48 hours and then gradually deflated and removed. If this fails other conservative surgical interventions such as Brace suture may be attempted, depending on clinical circumstances and available expertise.

Obstetric haemorrhage is a significant contributor to worldwide maternal morbidity and mortality, therefore definite protocol/ guidelines should be available in every labour ward and should be regularly updated. A stepwise escalation of pharmacological and eventual surgical approaches should be clearly written and kept on the labour ward all the time.

(Reference – RCOG Green-top guidelines no. 52)

EMQs on PPROM (Preterm Premature Rupture of Membranes), Prematurity and Prophylactic Steroid

Options for questions 17 – 18

A	Ultrasound examination and digital examination	F	Insulin-like growth factor binding protein-1
B	Sterile speculum examination	G	Digital vaginal examination
C	Nitrazine test	H	Amniocentesis
D	USG examination	I	Fetal fibronectin
E	Fern test	J	AmniSure

Instruction: For each question posed below, choose the single most appropriate answer from the A–J list above. The given option may be used once, more than once or not at all.

Question 17	An 18 year old primigravida at 32 weeks of pregnancy has attended the labour ward with a history of leaking fluid per vaginum for the past 4 hours. She has no pain or contractions and fetal movement is present.
Answer 17	
Question 18	A 26 year old second gravida complains of leaking per vagina for 4 days at 28 weeks of pregnancy. She describes a clear, watery gush of fluid intermittently. On speculum examination, leaking fluid could not be demonstrated. Initial inspection of pad remains dry.
Answer 18	

Answers and explanations

Answer 17 (B) Sterile speculum examination

The diagnosis of spontaneous rupture of the membranes is best achieved by maternal history followed by a sterile speculum examination.

Cervical swab including *Chlamydia trachomatis* and *Neisseria gonorrhoeae* and vaginal swab for *Streptococcus agalactiae* should be obtained if possible. Maternal vital signs should be documented regularly including temperature and pulse. Fetal monitoring with continuous CTG should be performed initially to establish fetal well-being.

Digital examination of the cervix with PPROM has been shown to shorten latency and increase the risk of infections without providing any additional useful clinical information. Visual inspection of the cervix can estimate cervical dilatation, however, it can be difficult in certain situation where the vaginal wall is floppy e.g. in parous women.

Answer 18 (D) Ultrasound examination

Ultrasound examination is useful in some cases to help confirm the diagnosis as it might demonstrate oligohydramnios where history is not helpful or clinical examination is inconclusive. Ultrasonographic documentation of gestational age, fetal weight, fetal presentation and amniotic fluid index should be established in these cases.

Options for questions 19 – 20

A	Consider therapeutic tocolysis	F	Amniocentesis to confirm fetal infection
B	Consider steroids	G	USG
C	Amnio infusion	H	Involve neonatologist
D	Consider delivery	I	Consider antibiotic
E	Transfer to fetal medicine centre	J	Consider prophylactic tocolysis

Instruction: For each question posed below, choose the single most appropriate management from the A-J list above. The given option may be used once, more than once or not at all.

Question 19	A 34 year old primigravida is complaining of leaking clear fluid for the past 5 hours per vagina at 32 weeks of gestation. SROM has been confirmed by speculum examination. She has no pain or contraction. However, she is recently feeling mild discomfort, which is similar to period-like pain. CTG of fetus shows non-reassuring fetal heart pattern.
Answer 19	
Question 20	A 36 year old in her second pregnancy complains of leaking clear fluid per vagina. She is currently 35 weeks pregnant and has had an uneventful pregnancy. She has no pain or contractions and is booked under midwife-led care.
Answer 20	

Answers and explanations

Answer 19 (D) Consider delivery

In this case, delivery is required as there is an abnormal CTG indicating fetal compromise.

Expectant management should be preferred if fetal and maternal well-being is normal and stable. The risks and potential benefits of expectant management should be discussed with the patient and her family, and informed consent should be obtained where appropriate.

The maternal and fetal status need to be reevaluated daily, and the safety and potential benefits of expectant management should be reassessed. The benefit of even a short period is important, to allow administration of steroids and antibiotics.

Once maturity has been reached, the benefit from expectant management of PPROM is unclear and the risks of infection outweigh any potential benefits after 34 weeks of gestation. However, there is no randomized control trial available to confirm the gestational age when the delivery should be expedited.

Answer 20 (D) Consider delivery (delivery should be considered at 34 weeks of gestation)

PPROM is a common complication of pregnancy occurring in about 3% of all pregnancies. The obstetrician needs to be familiar with appropriate management of PPROM and guidelines should be available in the delivery suite locally according to the availability of SCBU and the conservative management for antenatal monitoring.

Maternal health is the primary indicator for the need to deliver. Therefore, any evidence of infection or maternal instability (bleeding, temperature, lower abdominal pain) requires careful evaluation and appropriateness and determination of expectant management. After 34 weeks' gestation, the appropriateness of expectant management of PPROM should be reevaluated individually for each case.

Fetal monitoring with CTG should be performed at least daily until delivery, and fetal well-being and growth should be evaluated periodically (1–2 weeks) with ultrasonography.

Options for questions 21 – 23

A	Corticosteroid dose may be repeated	**H**	Corticosteroid may be used cautiously
B	Dexamethasone 12mg IM 24 hours apart	**I**	Benefits of steroid not clear
C	Betamethasone 24mg IM 24 hours apart	**J**	Dexamethasone 24mg IM stat
D	Betamethasone 12 mg IM 24 hours apart	**K**	Prophylactic steroid should be given
E	Oral Betamethasone 12mg 24 hours apart	**L**	Oral Dexamethasone 12mg 24 hours apart
F	Prevents more than 1% of respiratory problem in neonates	**M**	Prevents more than 60% of respiratory problem in neonates
G	Corticosteroids are contraindicated	**N**	No role of prophylactic steroid

Instruction: For each question posed below, choose the single most appropriate answer from the A-N list above. The given option may be used once, more than once or not at all.

Question 21	A 26 year old primigravida has preterm rupture of membranes at 32 weeks of gestation. She has been having pain and contraction for 5 hours of duration. She is suffering from tuberculosis, which has been diagnosed recently.
Answer 21	
Question 22	A 22 year old in second pregnancy has attended the labour ward with pain and contraction. She has been offered prophylactic steroid for fetal lung maturation. What is the most suitable and effective steroid regime for the woman?
Answer 22	
Question 23	A 38 year old primigravida visits the antenatal clinic and wants to discuss prophylactic corticosteroid at 30 weeks. She has conceived after IVF. USG scan has confirmed it to be Dichorionic Diamniotic twin pregnancy. She does not have pain or contraction.
Answer 23	

Answers and explanations

Answer 21 (H) Corticosteroid may be used cautiously

Corticosteroid therapy can suppress immune system further in pregnant woman and exacerbates infection. However, there is no evidence to suggest that a single course will have profound effect. During active infection it should be used with caution.

Answer 22 (D) Betamethasone 12mg IM 24 hours apart

Betamethasone is the steroid of choice to enhance lung maturation. Recommended therapy involves two doses of betamethasone 12mg, given intramuscularly 24 hours apart. Antenatal exposure to betamethasone is associated with a decreased risk of cystic periventricular leucomalacia among premature infants born at 24-31 weeks of gestation.

Comparison of oral versus intramuscular administration of dexamethasone suggests no difference in the frequency of RDS between the two modes of drug delivery. However, neonatal sepsis seems to be increased with oral dexamethasone.

Answer 23 (N) No role of prophylactic steroid

There is no evidence to support prophylactic steroids in multiple pregnancies. A retrospective cohort study demonstrated that a prophylactic approach of administering antenatal corticosteroids every two weeks from 24 to 32 weeks was not associated with a significant reduction in RDS.

Options for questions 24 – 26

A	Ritodrine	H	Glyceryl trinitrate
B	Nifedipine	I	Indomethacin
C	Atosiban	J	Reassurance
D	Postpone delivery till beds are available in SCBU	K	Deliver the baby and transfer to another hospital
E	Labour to be induced and in the meantime bed may become available in SCBU	L	Deliver the baby and need for transfer can be assessed after delivery
F	Isoxsuprine hydrochloride	M	Maintenance therapy cannot be recommended
G	Transfer to tertiary care	N	Magnesium sulphate

Instruction: For each option posed below, choose the single **most appropriate tocolysis** from the A-N list above. The given option may be used once, more than once or not at all.

Question 24	A 34 year old second gravida is admitted with threatened preterm labour at 30 weeks of gestation. She is contracting 3 in 10. Vaginal examination done shows os to be 1.5 cm dilated, and 50% effaced.
Answer 24	
Question 25	A 40 year old primigravida is admitted with threatened preterm labour at 26 weeks of gestation. She is contracting 4 in 10. Vaginal examination done shows os to be 2 cm dilated, and 30% effaced. There is no bed in SCBU.
Answer 25	
Question 26	A 36 year old primigravida is admitted at 33 weeks of gestation with severe pre-eclampsia. She is on methyldopa 500 qid and labetalol 200mg tds. Her blood pressure is 140/106 mmhg. She has got three plus proteinuria and she is complaining of a headache. There is no bed in SCBU.
Answer 26	

Answers and explanations

Answer 24 (C) Atosiban

Oxytocin antagonists are synthetic analogues that have the nonapeptide structure of oxytocin. They act by competing with oxytocin for receptors in the myometrium. Atosiban is significantly better tolerated than the beta2-agonists, particularly with regard to the cardiovascular side effects. Atosiban is licensed for this usage in the UK but nifedipine is not.

Answer 25 (G) Transfer to tertiary care

Tocolytic should be started to arrest labour and arrangement should be made for the transfer in-utero. Progressive cervical dilatation and effacement can be delayed, which may defer delivery for some time and the administration of steroid considered. It allows the mother to be brought to a specialized centre that is equipped and staffed to handle preterm deliveries.

Answer 26 (K) Deliver the baby and transfer to another hospital

The mother should be stabilized first and it is advisable to deliver the baby locally as the risk to the mother during the transferral is high. Ex-utero transfer should be considered for the safety of the mother and baby.

Options for questions 27 – 28

A	Palpitations	G	Pulmonary oedema
B	Tremor	H	Vomiting
C	Nausea	I	Dyspnoea
D	Headache	J	Tachycardia
E	Hypotension	K	Facial puffiness
F	Chest pain	L	Pedal oedema

Instruction: For each question posed below, choose the single most appropriate answer from the A–L list above. The given option may be used once, more than once not at all.

Question 27	A 27 year old primigravida is admitted with a 26 week pregnancy. She is contracting two in ten. Atosiban has been started. What is the most common side effect of it?
Answer 27	
Question 28	A 36 year old third gravida is admitted for external cephalic version. Tocolysis has been offered with GTN patch. What is the most common adverse effect of it?
Answer 28	

Answers and explanations

Answer 27 (C) Nausea

Compared to betamimetics, use of atosiban is associated with a significantly lower frequency of adverse events for tachycardia, palpitation, vomiting, headache, hyperglycaemia, tremor, dyspnoea, chest pain, hypocalemia and fetal tachycardia.

Answer 28 (D) Headache

The most common side effects are a throbbing headache, flushing and dizziness. These may occur as a result of vasodilatation. They are unpleasant, but not serious.

(Reference – RCOG Green-top guidelines nos.1B, 7 and 44)

EMQs on the Abnormal Attachment of Placenta and Umbilical Cord

Options for questions 29 – 32

A	TVS	**H**	X-ray
B	TVS at 32 weeks	**I**	Colour Doppler USG
C	CT scan	**J**	Reassurance
D	MRI at 32 weeks	**K**	TVS at 38 weeks
E	Three dimensional Power Doppler	**L**	Trans-abdominal scan at 28 weeks
F	Trans-abdominal scan at 30 weeks	**M**	MRI at 34 weeks
G	TVS at 36 weeks	**N**	MRI at 38 weeks

Instruction: For each question posed below, choose the single most appropriate answer from the list above. The given option may be used once, more than once or not at all.

Question 29	A primigravida had a routine anomaly scan at 22 weeks and was found to have low-lying placenta. She had spontaneous pregnancy and no risk factors have been identified. What further action should be taken?
Answer 29	
Question 30	A multigravida woman in her 4th pregnancy admitted with intermittent vaginal bleeding at 18 weeks. Placenta was found to be postero-lateral and difficult to visualize the lower edge. Transvaginal scan was performed after informed consent to localize the placenta and was found to cover the internal os completely.
Answer 30	
Question 31	A primigravida attended to her community midwife at 26 weeks for routine checkup. She had a history of spotting at 24 weeks, which settled without any intervention. She had an anomaly scan at 22 weeks, which had suggested a low-lying placenta. At that time a transvaginal scan was performed which had suggested minor placenta praevia.
Answer 31	
Question 32	A 30 year old woman in her third pregnancy had a routine anomaly scan at 21 weeks. The placenta was noted to be anterior and low-lying. She has previously had one vaginal delivery and one emergency caesarean section a year ago.
Answer 32	

Answers and explanations

Answer 29 (A) TVS

A transvaginal ultrasound scan should be recommended where low-lying placenta is suspected at the anomaly scan (20–22 weeks). It is significantly more accurate and safe. Sixty percent of women who undergo TAS may have a reclassification of placental location after TVS. This helps to reduce the numbers of those for whom follow-up will be needed to check the placental location.

In posteriorly situated placenta TAS is associated with 25% of false positive rate due to poor visualization. Fetal head, obesity and under or overfilling of the bladder often interferes in visualization of the lower segment.

Answer 30 (B) TVS at 32 weeks

In cases with asymptomatic suspected major placenta praevia (covering the cervical os), a transvaginal ultrasound scan should be performed at 32 weeks. This clarifies the diagnosis and allows planning for third trimester management and delivery.

It is not unusual to detect a low-lying placenta or to see the placenta covering the internal os during a routine mid pregnancy ultrasound. Most of these cases resolve themselves before late pregnancy (as the uterus grows the placenta migrates away).

If the placenta is completely covering the cervical os at an earlier scan, it is recommended that its position should be checked by TAS at 32 weeks. If the scan result is not clear, TVS should be performed.

Placental migration is less likely if the placenta is posterior, if there is a previous caesarean section scar or placenta praevia major is present.

Answer 31 (G) TVS at 36 weeks

In cases of asymptomatic suspected minor praevia, follow-up imaging can be left until 36 weeks.

Answer 32 (E) Three dimensional Power Doppler

Antenatal imaging by three dimensional (3D) Power Doppler should be performed in women with anterior placenta praevia who are at increased risk of placenta accreta. The sensitivity is 100% and specificity 85%.

The marked increase in the incidence of placenta accreta has been attributed to the increased prevalence of caesarean delivery in recent years.

Patients who are at risk should be identified as early as in the first trimester by an ultrasound examination. The characteristic findings include a low-lying sac that appears to be attached to the anterior uterine wall.

Irregular vascular sinuses appear as early as 16 weeks, which have turbulent flow within. The bladder wall may appear interrupted or have small bulges of the placenta into the bladder space. Absence of the normal echolucent space between the placenta and myometrium is not a reliable sign by itself, as this space may be absent in normally situated anterior placenta.

Options for questions 33 – 36

A	Elective caesarean section at 38-39 weeks	G	Caesarean hysterectomy
B	Emergency caesarean section	H	Admitted and managed as in-patient
C	Tocolysis	I	Vaginal delivery
D	She should attend hospital immediately	J	Uterine artery embolization
E	Blood transfusion	K	Reassurance
F	Cervical cerclage	L	MRI

Instruction: For each question posed below, choose the single most appropriate answer from the A–L list above. The given option may be used once, more than once or not at all.

Question 33	A 34 year old woman had been diagnosed to have major placenta praevia and is admitted in the antenatal ward with mild backache at 34 weeks' gestation. She is not bleeding. She requests a caesarean section at 36 weeks.
Answer 33	
Question 34	A 36 year old multigravida attended an antenatal clinic for the first time at 34 weeks of gestation. She had received her earlier antenatal care in a different hospital and moved house recently. She had one episode of bleeding at 26 weeks. She was diagnosed to have major placenta praevia at the anomaly scan and it was confirmed at 32 weeks.
Answer 34	
Question 35	A 29 year old woman is diagnosed to have placenta praevia at a routine anomaly scan. She does not like hospital and prefers to stay at home unless there is a need. She is complaining of vague suprapubic discomfort.
Answer 35	
Question 36	A 24 year old primigravida has had a growth scan for suspected small for dates. USG scan at 34 weeks shows placental edge less than 2 cm from the internal os, placenta is thick. She has never had any bleeding.
Answer 36	

Answers and explanations

Answer 33 (A) Elective caesarean section at 38–39 weeks

The timing of an emergency caesarean section is influenced by individual circumstances. However, elective caesarean section should be deferred until 38 weeks to minimise neonatal morbidity and respiratory problems due to prematurity.

The use of prophylactic steroid is always beneficial in case of earlier delivery before 36 weeks, in case of recurrent bleeding.

Answer 34 (H) Admitted and managed as in-patient

The patient with diagnosed placenta praevia major can bleed suddenly and heavily, which requires urgent delivery. Each episode of bleeding is heavier than before and usually happens in the night, therefore hospital admission is considered during the latter part of the third trimester (from 34 weeks).

In woman who remains asymptomatic proper counselling regarding hospital admission should be given. Home care can be considered at request from a woman who lives close to the hospital and has immediate transport available. Informed consent must be taken from such women.

Available studies have not shown any difference regarding maternal or fetal morbidity with home management versus hospitalisation, prior to the first bleed.

Answer 35 (D) She should attend hospital immediately

The woman who is being managed at home should attend hospital immediately if she experiences any bleeding, contractions or pain (including vague suprapubic period-like aches). These symptoms might be associated with contraction and effacement of cervix causing bleeding.

Answer 36 (A) Elective caesarean section at 38–39 weeks

The mode of delivery should be based on clinical judgment supplemented by sonographic information available. A placental edge less than 2 cm from the internal os is likely to need delivery by caesarean section, especially if it is thick.

Options for questions 37 – 38

A	Most likely diagnosis is scar pregnancy	**G**	Laparotomy should be considered
B	Most likely it is cervical pregnancy	**H**	Hysterectomy is the best option
C	Internal iliac artery ligation should be performed	**I**	Repeat scan should be performed at 12 weeks
D	Methotrexate should be injected	**J**	Pregnancy should be terminated at once
E	Suction evacuation should not be performed	**K**	Angular implantation of gestational sac
F	Immediate laparoscopy is indicated	**L**	Interstitial implantation

Instruction: For each question posed below, choose the single most appropriate answer from the A–L list above. The given option may be used once, more than once or not at all.

Question 37	A 28 year woman in her second pregnancy is admitted with dull aching abdominal pain and mild vaginal bleeding. She has had an emergency caesarean section for failure to progress in the second stage of labour two years ago. On USG scan pregnancy found to be implanted very low in the lower segment. The pregnancy is corresponding to 7 weeks of gestation. Fetal heartbeat was present. There was absence of normal myometrium in between bladder and sac.
Answer 37	
Question 38	A 38 year old woman has presented in the early pregnancy unit with spotting and discomfort in the lower abdomen. She has had two therapeutic abortions in the early second trimester and one caesarean section. The gestation sac was found to be in the cervical canal with live fetus corresponding to 8 weeks' gestation.
Answer 38	

Answers and explanations

Answer 37 (A) Most likely diagnosis is scar pregnancy

In scar pregnancy the gestation sac is completely surrounded by myometrium and the fibrous tissue of the caesarean section scar, separated from the endometrial cavity and endocervical canal. More caesarean scar pregnancies are seen nowadays, probably because more and more deliveries are done by CS.

The diagnosis is usually made on ultrasonography revealing (1) an empty uterine cavity and an empty cervical canal (2) a gestational sac in the anterior part of the uterine isthmus and (3) an absence of healthy myometrium between the bladder and sac.

Expectant management of a viable scar pregnancy puts the mother at significant risk of an emergency hysterectomy if the pregnancy progresses beyond the first trimester.

Answer 38 (B) Most likely it is cervical pregnancy

Cervical pregnancy is a rare form of ectopic pregnancy in which the pregnancy implants in the lining of the endocervical canal. It accounts for less than 1% of ectopic pregnancies. On speculum examination, the external os may be open, revealing fetal membranes or pregnancy tissue, which appear blue or purple. The success of conservative treatment for cervical pregnancy depends on the diagnostic accuracy of the initial ultrasound. Correct diagnosis reduces the chance of hysterectomy or blood transfusion. Cervical pregnancies can be successfully managed without surgical intervention through local injection of methotrexate and KCl. This treatment not only ablates the ectopic pregnancy but also preserves the uterus for subsequent pregnancies. The conservative management is effective and safe.

Options for questions 39 – 41

A	LSCS as soon as possible	G	Admit to the ward
B	Advise termination of pregnancy	H	Routine antenatal care
C	Imaging should be repeated in third trimester	I	MRI to confirm the diagnosis
D	Should be sent to fetal medicine unit	J	Antenatal care weekly
E	LSCS in between 35–37 weeks	K	Vaginal delivery can be allowed
F	LSCS at 39 weeks	L	Repeat scan weekly

Instruction: For each question posed below, choose the single most appropriate answer from the A–L list above. The given option may be used once, more than once or not at all.

Question 39	A 30 year old primigravida was admitted with bleeding per vaginum at 20 weeks of gestation. Ultrasound scan performed suspected low-lying placenta and vasa praevia.
Answer 39	
Question 40	A 26 year old second gravida has come to the antenatal clinic at 30 weeks of gestation. She had a scan done 2 days ago and it has confirmed vasa praevia.
Answer 40	
Question 41	A 29 year old second gravida is admitted in the ward at 32 weeks of gestation. Vasa previa has been confirmed on the scan. She has had two previous vaginal deliveries. This pregnancy has so far been uncomplicated. Mode of delivery is being discussed.
Answer 41	

Answers and explanations

Answer 39 (C) Imaging should be repeated in third trimester

Vasa praevia is present when fetal vessels traverse the lower uterine segments in advance of the presenting part. It may be suspected when an antenatal sonogram with colour-flow Doppler reveals a vessel crossing the membranes over the internal cervical os.

As gestation advances vasa praevia can resolve in up to 15% of cases. Therefore, it is essential to confirm persistence of vasa previa in the third trimester as delivery can then be planned.

Answer 40 (G) Admit to the ward

Once vasa praevia is confirmed the woman should be offered admission from 28 to 32 weeks of gestation. This allows quick intervention if required.

Answer 41 (E) LSCS in between 35–37 weeks

Elective LSCS is planned between 35–37 weeks of pregnancy when risk of prematurity significantly decreases. Spontaneous labour should be avoided as it will lead to tearing of blood vessels and fetal haemorrhage, leading to death.

(Reference – RCOG Green-top guideline no.27)

EMQs on External Cephalic Version and Breech Presentation

Options for questions 42 – 43

A	10%	F	20%
B	40%	G	30%
C	50%	H	60%
D	70%	I	80%
E	90%	J	100%

Instruction: For each question posed below, choose the single most appropriate answer from the A–J list above. The given option may be used once, more than once or not at all.

Question 42	A 32 year old multigravida has come at 37 weeks with breech presentation. She is about to consent to external cephalic version. She wants to know the overall success rate of external cephalic version.
Answer 42	
Question 43	A 26 year old primigravida has come for an antenatal checkup at 34 weeks. It is found that presentation is breech. She is being offered external cephalic version. She wants to know the success rate.
Answer 43	

Answers and explanations

Answer 42 (H) 60%

At 32 weeks' gestation, approximately 16% of fetuses are in the breech position. This rate decreases to 3–4% at term. Data suggests that the chance of spontaneous version after 36 weeks is only 5–8%. A wide range of success rates for external cephalic version is reported in the literature.

Institutions routinely offering external cephalic version have success rates ranging from 35% to 76%. An overall success rate of 60% for multiparous woman can usually be achieved.

External cephalic version has been shown to decrease the number of breech births as well as decrease the rate of caesarean delivery.

Answer 43 (B) 40%

ECV should be done at 36 weeks in primigravida. An overall success rate of 40% for nulliparous woman can be achieved. ECV is a valuable though underused option in the management of breech presentation at term. It is a relatively safe procedure, simple to learn and perform.

Vigilance for breech presentation after 34 weeks is important. A proper understanding of the risk is essential for the obstetrician to allow accurate counselling. All well-equipped obstetric units should offer ECV to suitable women at or near term with breech and other malpresentations.

Options for questions 44 – 45

A	30 weeks	F	28 weeks
B	32 weeks	G	26 weeks
C	34 weeks	H	37 weeks
D	35 weeks	I	39 weeks
E	36 weeks	J	38 weeks

Instruction: For each question posed below, choose the single **most appropriate gestational age to do ECV** from the A–J list above. The given option may be used once, more than once or not at all.

Question 44	A 32 year old primigravida attended for ANC checkup with the community midwife at 34 weeks' gestation. Presentation is found to be breech, which was confirmed by USG scan. External cephalic version was discussed and agreed.
Answer 44	
Question 45	A third gravida with two previous normal deliveries attended ANC checkup at 36 weeks. USG scan confirms extended breech presentation. External cephalic version was discussed and agreed.
Answer 45	

Answers and explanations

Answer 44 (E) ECV should be offered from 36 weeks in nulliparous women

Answer 45 (H) ECV should be offered from 37 weeks in multiparous women

ECV before 36 weeks of gestation is not associated with a significant reduction in breech births.

In primigravida, ECV should be offered from 36 weeks.
There is no upper time limit on the appropriate gestation for ECV.

Options for questions 46 – 48

A	Instrumental delivery	G	Episiotomy
B	Fetal blood sampling from the buttocks	H	External cephalic version
C	Radiological pelvimetry	I	Fundal pressure
D	Vaginal birth is contraindicated	J	Labour augmentation with oxytocin
E	Emergency caesarean section	K	Ultrasound to confirm the presentation
F	Epidural analgesia	L	Breech extraction

Instruction: For each question posed below, choose the single most appropriate answer from the A–L list above. The given option may be used once, more than once or not at all.

Question 46	A 36 year old third gravida has opted for vaginal breech birth. She had one previous vaginal breech delivery three years ago. During labour there is delay in the descent of the breech in the second stage of labour.
Answer 46	
Question 47	A third gravida has come for antenatal checkup at 36 weeks of gestation. Breech presentation is suspected, which is confirmed by USG scan. She wants a vaginal breech delivery. Caesarean section was done two years ago for a failure to progress of labour.
Answer 47	
Question 48	A fourth gravida has come to the labour ward for external cephalic version at 39 weeks of gestation. She has had previously three normal deliveries. CTG done revealed that she is regularly contracting. She was booked for ECV one week ago.
Answer 48	

Answers and explanations

Answer 46 (E) Emergency caesarean section

Failure of the presenting part to descend may be a sign of relative cephalopelvic disproportion. Caesarean section should be considered.

Answer 47 (D) Vaginal birth is contraindicated

Factors regarded as unfavorable for vaginal breech birth include the following:

- placenta praevia
- compromised fetal condition
- clinically inadequate pelvis
- footling or kneeling breech presentation
- large baby (usually defined as larger than 3800g)
- growth-restricted baby (usually defined as smaller than 2000g)
- hyperextended fetal neck in labour (diagnosed with ultrasound or X-ray where ultrasound is not available)
- previous caesarean section
- lack of presence of a clinician trained in vaginal breech delivery.

Answer 48 (K) Ultrasound to confirm the presentation

ECV can be offered at the onset of labour if membranes are intact, but as she was booked one week ago, presentation should be confirmed first by scan.

(Reference – RCOG Green-top guidelines nos. 20a, 20b)

EMQs on Infectious Disease in Pregnancy

Options for questions 49 – 53

A	Intrapartum prophylaxis with oral clindamycin 600mg eight hourly to be considered	**H**	Intrapartum prophylaxis with IV clindamycin 900mg eight hourly to be considered
B	Antenatal screening and prophylaxis e.g. urine culture and high vaginal swab culture is recommended from 36 weeks of pregnancy	**I**	Intrapartum prophylaxis with penicillin G 3gm IV followed by 1.5gm every 4 hourly
C	High vaginal swab culture for group B streptococcal infection from 36 weeks onwards	**J**	Antenatal penicillin injection every month from 16 weeks of pregnancy
D	Urine culture for group B streptococcal infection from 36 weeks onwards	**K**	Antenatal screening and prophylaxis is not recommended
E	Intrapartum prophylaxis with intravenous erythromycin 500mg every 4 hourly to be considered	**L**	No need for intrapartum prophylaxis
F	Intrapartum prophylaxis with penicillin G 9gm IV followed by 3gm every 4 hourly	**M**	Intrapartum prophylaxis with penicillin G 1.5gm every 4 hourly
G	Intrapartum prophylaxis with penicillin G6 gm IV followed by 3gm every 4 hourly	**N**	Intrapartum prophylaxis with oral erythromycin 500mg every 4 hourly to be considered

Instruction: For each question posed below, choose the single most appropriate answer from the list above. The given option may be used once, more than once or not at all.

Question 49	A 30 year old second gravida at 10 weeks has come for an antenatal checkup. It is noticed that her previous baby had group B steptococcal infection at birth and was admitted in special care baby unit for 10 days. She is anxious and wants to know about antenatal measures.
Answer 49	
Question 50	A 26 year old primigravida is admitted in labour at 34 weeks of pregnancy. She is complaining of leaking per vaginum since the last 20 hours. On examination, she is afebrile. Fetus is in cephalic presentation and on vaginal examination cervix is 4 cm dilated, 50% effaced and vertex is at 0 station.
Answer 50	
Question 51	A 32 year old third gravida is admitted in labour at 38 weeks of pregnancy. She is complaining of leaking per vaginum since last 24 hours. On examination, she is febrile and her pulse is 106/ minute. Uterus is not tender and fetal heart rate is 156/minute. On vaginal examination cervix is 2 cm dilated, 80% effaced and vertex is at -2 station. She is allergic to penicillin.
Answer 51	
Question 52	A 36 year old second gravida is admitted for induction of labour at 37 weeks due to severe pregnancy-induced hypertension. Her previous baby had died due to severe group B streptococcal infection at birth.
Answer 52	

Question 53	A 37 year old primigravida is admitted at 37 weeks with labour pain. While reviewing her antenatal notes it is found that she had urinary tract infection at 24 weeks. Group B steptococcus was detected in urine when the culture was repeated at 26 weeks.
Answer 53	

Answers and explanations

Answer 49 (K) Antenatal screening and prophylaxis is not recommended

Group B *Streptococcus* (GBS) is a part of normal flora of the gut and genital tract and is found in 20–40% women. It may be harmful to both mother and the baby and result in neonatal death due to severe neonatal infection.

Routine screening (either bacteriological or risk based) for antenatal GBS carriage is not recommended. Antenatal treatment with penicillin is not recommended.

Answer 50 (I) Intrapartum prophylaxis with penicillin G 3gm IV followed by 1.5gm every 4 hourly

In the UK, women are treated according to their risk in labour – antibiotics are given to:

- women whose membranes are ruptured for more than 18 hours
- those who have fever
- prematurity < 37 weeks
- previous baby with neonatal GBS disease
- if GBS is detected incidentally in the vagina or the urine in the current pregnancy.

Treatment of GBS-carrier mothers with the above risk factors during labour lead to a 60% reduction in neonatal infection rate and 95% reduction in neonatal death.

Penicillin G as prophylaxis should be administered as soon as possible after the onset of labour and at least 2 hours before delivery.

Answer 51 (H) Intrapartum prophylaxis with IV clindamycin 900mg 8 hourly to be considered

Answer 52 (I) Intrapartum prophylaxis with penicillin G 3gm IV followed by 1.5gm every 4 hourly

Answer 53 (I) Intrapartum prophylaxis with penicillin G 3gm IV followed by 1.5gm every 4 hourly

Options for questions 54 – 56

A	Viral culture is not recommended	G	Type specific HSV antibody testing
B	Caesarean section	H	Vaginal delivery
C	Referred to a genitourinary physician	I	Rupture of membranes should be avoided
D	Viral culture during last six weeks	J	Suppressive acyclovir is not recommended
E	Intravenous acyclovir	K	Oral acyclovir
F	Rupture of membranes should be avoided and intravenous acyclovir to be given	L	Suppressive acyclovir 500mg thrice daily from 36 weeks of gestation

Instruction: For each question posed below, choose the single **most appropriate initial management** from the above list above. The given option may be used once, more than once or not at all.

Question 54	A 20 year old primigravida at 22 weeks of gestation notices some painful vesicles at her gentiles. GP surgery suspects it to be genital herpes. This is her first episode.
Answer 54	
Question 55	A 30 year old third gravida has her first episode of genital herpes infection at 35^{+2} weeks of gestation. She has had two previous normal deliveries. She is unwilling for LSCS and has opted for vaginal delivery.
Answer 55	
Question 56	A 36 year old primigravida was diagnosed to have genital herpes at 22 weeks of gestation. It was her first episode. But she is very anxious and is discussing suppressive therapy to prevent recurrence of lesions at term as she is keen to have vaginal delivery.
Answer 56	

Answers and explanations

Answer 54 (C) Referred to a genitourinary physician

The main concern with maternal herpes simplex virus (HSV) infection during pregnancy is the risk of neonatal infection. This can lead to severe neurological impairment and to death. Neonatal herpes occurs in fewer than 2 per 100,000 live births. It usually results from maternal viral shedding during delivery, which may be asymptomatic. It may also rarely be acquired in-utero. If it is the first episode, referral to genitourinary medicine should be made where confirmation of the diagnosis (by viral culture or polymerase chain reaction), advice on management and screening for other sexually transmitted infections can be arranged.

Answer 55 (F) Rupture of membranes should be avoided and intravenous acyclovir to be given

Caesarean section is recommended for women who develop primary genital herpes within 6 weeks of delivery. If they opt for vaginal delivery, rupture of membranes and invasive procedures should be avoided. Intravenous acyclovir for the mother intrapartum and for the neonate after birth should be considered.

Answer 56 (J) Suppressive acyclovir is not recommended

Regular viral swabs and culture in late pregnancy do not predict viral shedding at term and are not recommended. If the woman has a history of recurrent genital herpes, she should be reassured that the risk of transmitting the infection to her baby is very small (even if she does have active lesions at delivery). Similarly, there is insufficient evidence to recommend use of daily suppressive acyclovir from 36 weeks of gestation to prevent recurrence of lesion.

Options for questions 57 – 62

A	Blood test for confirmation of VZV immunity	F	Should attend A&E immediately
B	A careful history for significance and susceptibility of infection	G	A hospital assessment should be considered
C	Reassurance	H	VZIG as soon as possible
D	Oral acyclovir	I	IV acyclovir
E	Amoxicillin and oral acyclovir	J	Notify their doctor or midwife

Instruction: For each question posed below, choose the single most appropriate answer from the A–J list above. The given option may be used once, more than once or not at all.

Question 57	A 32 year school teacher is currently 10 weeks pregnant for the first time. She is very anxious as she came in contact with a child who had chickenpox. She seeks an appointment with her GP.
Answer 57	
Question 58	A 26 year old woman in her second pregnancy at twelve weeks has visited her GP. Her daughter has developed chickenpox. She is not sure about her past infection and her immunity status is not known.
Answer 58	
Question 59	A primigravida at 12 weeks of pregnancy came in contact with a child who had chickenpox a week ago. She had received VZIG 3 days ago. She has noticed a rash on her forearm.
Answer 59	
Question 60	A 28 year old in her first pregnancy at 11 weeks was in contact with chickenpox infection in a nursery. A serum test done to find susceptibility to infection confirmed immunity to chickenpox.
Answer 60	
Question 61	A 26 year old second gravida has reported to her GP as she has contact with chickenpox infection 2 days ago. She is 16 weeks pregnant. Serum test done to find susceptibility of infection and found to be non immune.
Answer 61	
Question 62	A 32 year old third gravida has visited GP as she noticed rash on her legs. She has visited her sister 10 days ago. Her sister's son had chickenpox, which was confirmed by a general practitioner. She is 20 weeks pregnant.
Answer 62	

Answers and explanations

Answer 57 (B) A careful history for significance and susceptibility of infection

Infection in pregnancy is particularly likely to be complicated. If a pregnant woman reports contact with chickenpox, an attempt should be made to ascertain a history of previous infection to confirm the significance of the contact and the susceptibility of the patient as immunity might be assured.

80–85% of adults have had chickenpox in childhood. The remaining 15% are more likely to develop complications if they have chickenpox as an adult. Complications of chickenpox include pneumonitis, haemorrhagic chickenpox and encephalitis. Mortality and morbidity is very high, mostly due to pneumonitis.

Answer 58 (A) Blood test for confirmation of VZV immunity

If the history remains uncertain, the antibody status can be confirmed serologically. This may have to be repeated to see the appearance of IgM if titre is not confirmatory. The case should be discussed with the consultant microbiologist and serum antiody should be checked for confirmation of VZV immunity.

Answer 59 (J) Notify their doctor or midwife

Women who have had exposure to chickenpox or shingles (regardless of whether or not they have received VZIG) should notify their doctor or midwife early if a rash develops for further management.

Answer 60 (C) Reassurance

The presence of VZV immunoglobulin (IgG) antibody in the serum is indicative of immunity acquired from previous exposure. Therefore, the pregnant woman and her fetus are protected.

Answer 61 (H) VZIG as soon as possible

If the pregnant woman is seronegative and she has had a significant exposure, she should be given VZIG as soon as possible. It is effective when given up to 10 days after contact and becomes less useful with an increasing time interval. If not given within 10 days since contact then it has a little value and is less protective.

The rationale for offering VZIG is the potential protection offered to the mother, who has a high risk of severe complicated disease such as pneumonitis or meningitis.

Answer 62 (G) A hospital assessment should be considered

Risk of complication is high if the woman:

- smokes
- suffers from bronchitis or emphysema
- is taking or have taken steroids during the previous three months
- is more than 20 weeks pregnant.

10% pregnant women with chickenpox can develop pneumonia. Other rare complications include inflammation of other parts of the body, such as:

- encephalitis
- liver hepatitis

- myocarditis
- glomerulonephritis
- appendicitis
- pancreatitis.

Very rarely, complications from chickenpox during pregnancy can be fatal. Therefore, hospital assessment should be considered, even in the absence of immediate complications. Appropriate treatment should be decided after consultation with a multidisciplinary team: obstetrician, fetal medicine specialist, virologist and neonatologist

(Reference – RCOG Green-top guideline no.13)

Options for questions 63 – 66

A	Elective caesarean section at 38 weeks	H	Elective caesarean section at 39 weeks
B	Breastfeeding is contraindicated	I	Vaginal delivery is absolutely contraindicated
C	HAART should be initiated between 20-28 weeks and discontinued at delivery	J	Neonate should be given antiretroviral therapy within four hours of birth
D	HAART regimen should be continued throughout pregnancy and postpartum	K	HAART should be initiated between 10-12 weeks and discontinued at delivery
E	Urgent HIV test	L	Instrumental delivery
F	Patient with low viral load can breast feed their babies	M	Zidouvidine (ZDV) as monotherapy is not recommended now
G	Vaginal delivery can be offered	N	Zidouvidine (ZDV) monotherapy

Instruction: For each question posed below, choose the single most appropriate answer from the A–N list above. The given option may be used once, more than once or not at all.

Question 63	A 36 year old primigravida is 36 weeks pregnant. She is HIV positive and is on HAART (highly active antiretroviral therapy). Plasma viral load is 70 copies/ml. She is clinically asymptomatic and wants to discuss the mode of delivery.
Answer 63	
Question 64	A 34 year old third gravida is 38 weeks pregnant. She was diagnosed to be HIV positive in this pregnancy and is on HAART (highly active antiretroviral therapy). Plasma viral load is 20 copies/ml. She is clinically asymptomatic and wants to discuss the mode of delivery. She has had two previous normal vaginal deliveries. She is keen to have vaginal delivery.
Answer 64	
Question 65	A 29 year old primigravida is 38 weeks pregnant. She is HIV positive and on HAART. Her plasma viral load is 20 copies/ml. She is clinically asymptomatic and requesting a caesarean section.
Answer 65	
Question 66	A 36 year old HIV positive woman is 10 weeks pregnant. She does not require HAART for her own health. She wants to discuss measures regarding preventing maternal-to-child transmission. Her plasma viral load is 7000 copies/ml.
Answer 66	

Answers and explanations

Answer 63 (A) Elective caesarean section at 38 weeks

Indication for elective caesarean section in HIV woman as described below are:

- women taking HAART who have a plasma viral load greater than 50 copies/ml
- women taking ZDV monotherapy as an alternative to HAART
- women with HIV and hepatitis C virus co-infection.

Answer 64 (G) Vaginal delivery can be offered

All pregnant women should have their HIV serostatus evaluated at the antenatal booking. The risk of vertical transmission is as high as 25–30% without any treatment. The greatest risk of vertical transmission is thought to be advanced maternal disease and high maternal HIV viral load.

In addition to the standard prenatal assessment, continued assessment of HIV status is important. Initial evaluation includes CD4 counts, which help determine the degree of immunodeficiency. Viral load (determined by plasma HIV RNA copy number/mL) assesses the risk of disease progression.

As such, antiretroviral therapy should be offered to all pregnant women infected with HIV to reduce the risk of perinatal transmission.

Mother-to-child transmission rates can be reduced from 25–30% to less than 1% with antiretroviral therapy and avoidance of breastfeeding. Elective caesarean section in cases of high viral load and women on monotherapy can further reduce the risk of transmission.

If the patient presents to prenatal care on a HAART regimen, treatment should be continued. However, medication, which is contraindicated in pregnancy, should be avoided during the first trimester.

As zidouvidine (ZDV) is the only agent specifically shown to reduce perinatal transmission, it should be used as a part of the highly active antiretroviral therapy (HAART) regimen.

In women on HAART and with plasma viral loads of less than 50 copies/ml, vaginal delivery can be recommended. In these women, there is low risk of transmission to their babies.

Answer 65 (H) Elective caesarean section at 39 weeks

Elective caesarean sections should be performed at 39 completed weeks to reduce the chance of respiratory problem in neonates if it is done for maternal request or obstetric indications.

Answer 66 (C) HAART should be initiated between 20–28 weeks and discontinued at delivery

HAART should be initiated between 20 and 28 weeks and discontinued at delivery when given to minimise the risk of transmission. HAART regimen should be continued throughout pregnancy and postpartum when used for maternal health.

Options for questions 67 – 69

A	Admit to ICU	F	Chloroquine
B	IV quinine	G	Oral primaquine
C	IV primaquine	H	Reassurance
D	Admit to hospital	I	IV artesunate
E	IV quinine and clindamycin	J	Discontinue oral therapy

Instruction: For each question posed below, choose the single most appropriate management from the A–J list above. The given option may be used once, more than once or not at all.

Question 67	A 32 year old primigravida has come with a fever and has been vomiting for the last 3 days. She is 28 weeks pregnant. She is investigated for malaria. Her thick and thin smear shows more than 2% of red cells being parasitized.
Answers 67	
Question 68	A 30 year old woman has come with fever, prostation and lethargy. She is 20 weeks pregnant. She has recently visited a sub-Saharan country. Her thick and thin smear shows less than 2% of red cells being parasitized.
Answer 68	
Question 69	A 26 year old third gravida has come with fever. She has recently visited a sub-Saharan country. She is investigated for malaria. The tests done confirm *P. ovale* malaria.
Answer 69	

Answers and explanations

Answer 67 (A) Admit to ICU

Malaria is more common in pregnant women compared with the general population. Immunosuppression and loss of acquired immunity to malaria could be the causes. Due to the hormonal and immunological changes, the parasitemia tends to be 10 times higher and as a result, all the complications are more common in pregnancy compared to the non-pregnant population.

As *P. falciparum* malaria in pregnancy is more severe, the mortality is also double (13%) compared to the non-pregnant population (6.5%). The morbidity includes anaemia, fever illness, hypoglycemia, cerebral malaria, pulmonary edema and puerperal sepsis. Maternal mortality occurs from severe malaria and haemorrhage. The problems in the newborn include low birth weight, prematurity, IUGR and mortality.

Malaria in pregnancy should be treated as an emergency and should be admitted to an intensive care unit. Pregnant women with 2% or more parasitised red blood cells are at higher risk of developing severe malaria.

Answer 68 (D) Admit to hospital

Uncomplicated malaria in the UK is defined as fewer than 2% parasitised red blood cells in a woman with no signs of severity and no complicating features. They should be admitted to hospital for observation and treatment.

Answer 69 (F) Chloroquine

Chloroquine is the most effective medication for preventing and treating a malaria infection caused by *P. ovale*, *P. malariae*, or *P. knowlesi* parasites. It destroys the malarial parasite once it enters the bloodstream. As a prophylaxis, it should be taken for 4 weeks after leaving the area where malaria is present.

The lysosomotropic character of chloroquine is believed to account for much of its antimalarial activity. The drug concentrates in the acidic food vacuole of the parasite and interferes with essential processes. Chloroquine and related quinines have been associated with cases of retinal toxicity, particularly when provided at higher doses for longer time frames. Accumulation of the drug may result in deposits that can lead to blurred vision and blindness.

Options for questions 70 – 72

A	Start parenteral therapy	G	Oral primaquine
B	Oral chloroquine	H	Discontinue oral therapy
C	IV primaquine	I	IV artesunate
D	Give metoclopramide	J	Reassurance
E	IV quinine and clindamycin	K	Oral quinine and clindamycin
F	IV chloroquine	L	Oral artesunate

Instruction: For each question posed below, choose the single **most appropriate antimalarial** from the A–J list above. The given option may be used once, more than once or not at all.

Question 70	A 32 year old primigravida has come with fever, vomiting for the last 2 days at 28 weeks of pregnancy. Her thick and thin smear shows more than 2% of red cells being parasitized. She is admitted to ICU. Her tests done confirm *P. falciparum* malaria.
Answer 70	
Question 71	A 30 year old woman has come with fever for five days. She has recently visited a sub-Saharan country. She is 10 weeks pregnant. Malaria is suspected. Her thick and thin smear shows less than 2% of red cells being parasitized. She is admitted to hospital. Her tests done confirm *P. falciparum* malaria.
Answer 71	
Question 72	A 20 year old primigravida has come from Bangladesh. She c/o of fever, chills, headache and vomiting since 2 days. On examination, her temperature is raised and she is pale. Tests done confirmed *P. ovale* malaria. Oral chloroquine was started. She cannot tolerate oral therapy.
Answer 72	

Answers and explanations

Answer 70 (I) Intravenous artesunate

Intravenous artesunate is the treatment of choice for severe *falciparum* malaria. Intravenous quinine should be used as an alternative if artesunate is not available. The artemisinins produce rapid clearance of parasitaemia and therefore the rapid resolution of symptoms. It reduces parasite numbers 100- to 1000-fold per asexual cycle, which is more than the other currently available antimalarials.

Answer 71 (E) Intravenous quinine and clindamycin

Antimalarial medicines considered safe in the first trimester of pregnancy are quinine, chloroquine, clindamycin and proguanil.

Primaquine and tetracyclines should not be used in pregnancy. Quinine plus clindamycin for seven days (and quinine monotherapy if clindamycin is not available) can be used in uncomplicated *falciparum* malaria.

Answer 72 (D) Give metoclopramide

Vomiting is a symptom of malaria and a side effect of quinine, which may lead to treatment failure. Therefore, antiemetic should be used in combination. Metoclopramide is considered safe, in the first trimester.

After the antiemetic has had time to take effect, the dose should be repeated. Repeated vomiting after an antiemetic is an indication for parenteral therapy.

(Reference – RCOG Green-top guidelines nos. 13, 30, 36, 39, 54 A & B)

EMQs on Medical Disorders in Pregnancy

Options for questions 73 – 75

A	Peak anti-Xa activity	**F**	Ultrasound to be repeated in 2 weeks
B	D-dimer testing	**G**	Thrombophilia screen
C	Ultrasound to be repeated in 1 week	**H**	Compression duplex ultrasound
D	Magnetic resonance venography	**I**	Computed tomography pulmonary angiogram
E	A ventilation/perfusion (V/Q) lung scan	**J**	Chest X-ray

Instruction: For each question posed below, choose the single **most appropriate initial investigation** answer from the A–J list above. The given option may be used once, more than once or not at all.

Question 73	A 36 year old third gravida at 8 weeks has visited her general practitioner complaining of unilateral leg oedema and pain since last 3 days. She has had two uncomplicated pregnancies and spontaneous vaginal delivery at term. Recently her mother died of cerebrovascular accident at the age of 58.
Answer 73	
Question 74	A 30 year second gravida at 8 weeks has come complaining of leg oedema and pain since the last 3 days. On examination, both legs are tender, swollen and red. Low molecular weight heparin has been started and compression duplex USG advised. Her compression dulpex USG is negative. She is still symptomatic.
Answer 74	
Question 75	A 35 year old third gravida has presented as an emergency with chest pain and breathlessness since last 1 hour. She is 10 weeks pregnant and her BMI is 34. She is a known to have antithrombin 3 deficiencies and she was on warfarin. She stopped warfarin a year ago.
Answer 75	

Answers and explanations

Answer 73 (H) Compression duplex ultrasound

Real-time B-mode ultrasonography is the mainstay of objective investigation. The most reliable ultrasound criterion for thrombosis is a failure to collapse the vascular lumen completely with gentle probe pressure.

The sensitivity for duplex ultrasound for proximal thrombi is approximately 95%, and the specificity is 99%.

Answer 74 (C) Ultrasound to be repeated in 1 week

If diagnosis of DVT is confirmed by ultrasound, anticoagulant treatment should be continued. If the ultrasound is negative and clinical suspicion is high the woman should remain anticoagulated and ultrasound repeated in 1 week, or an alternative diagnostic test should be carried out.

Answer 75 (J) Chest X-ray

Signs and symptoms of PE are more problematic because dyspnea and tachypnea are common in pregnancy. In non-pregnant patients, tachypnea, dyspnea, chest pain (pleuritic), apprehension, and crackles are present in at least 50% of patients.

Chest radiographs are abnormal in 80% or more of patients with PE, and the findings are nonspecific. If there is a clinical suspicion of a PE, a chest X-ray should be organised. If this is normal, a compression duplex Doppler should be arranged. The chest X-ray may identify other pulmonary disease such as pneumonia, pneumothorax or lobar collapse. If the X-ray is abnormal with a high clinical suspicion of PTE, CTPA should be performed.

Options for questions 76 – 78

A	Platelet count	G	Thoracotomy
B	Intravenous unfractionated heparin	H	Oral anticoagulants
C	LMWH	I	Thrombolytic therapy
D	Surgical embolectomy	J	Plasma lipids
E	Full blood count	K	Factor v Leiden
F	D-dimer testing	L	Antithrombin III

Instruction: For each question posed below, choose the single most appropriate answer from the A–L list above. The given option may be used once, more than once or not at all.

Question 76	A 36 year old woman has come to A&E in a collapsed state. Her BMI is 34 and she has a family history of pulmonary embolism.
Answer 76	
Question 77	A 35 year old woman has presented in A&E with chest pain and dyspnoea. She is 10 weeks pregnant and her BMI is 34.
Answer 77	
Question 78	A 32 year old woman has had IVF pregnancy. She had developed hyperstimulation syndrome and needs admission to the hospital. Both her ovaries are enlarged and have developed ascites.
Answer 78	

Answers and explanations

Answer 76 (B) Intravenous unfractionated heparin

Heparin is an extensively used drug in the acute management of VTE, particularly massive PE with cardiovascular compromise. It is initiated with a loading dose of 5000 international units (IU) followed by a continuous infusion of 1000–2000 IU/hour depending on APTT measurements (at least daily), the first of which is taken 6 hours post loading dose. Prolonged unfractionated heparin use during pregnancy may result in osteoporosis and fractures.

Answer 77 (C) LMWH

If PE or DVT is strongly suspected then LMWH should be started as soon as possible unless it is contraindicated. The treatment should be continued until the diagnosis is excluded. LMWHs are as effective as unfractionated heparin for treatment of PE. The exact dose depends on the manufacturer's recommendations based on maternal pre-pregnancy weight and should be administered subcutaneously. There should be clear local guidelines for the dosage of LMWH to be used.

Oral anticoagulants cross the placenta readily and are associated with a characteristic embryopathy in the first trimester. Central nervous system abnormalities, which occur during any trimester, fetal and neonatal haemorrhage following the trauma of delivery, can occur easily.

Answer 78 (C) LMWH

For all women hospitalised with OHSS, prophylactic measures to prevent thromboembolic complications should be taken. If there is a personal or family history of thromboembolic events, thrombophilia, or vascular anomalies, thromboprophylaxsis is strongly recommended. Intermittent pneumatic compression device, stocking or heparin is recommended when a patient is confined to bed. If the woman does not conceive, and OHSS is resolving, it can be stopped.

If the woman conceives during the prophylaxis the risk of thrombosis persists in the first trimester and beyond. Therefore consideration should be given for continuation after discussion of the risks and benefits with the woman.

Options for questions 79 – 80

A	LMHW for 4 weeks postpartum	F	Unfractionated heparin
B	Therapeutic low molecular weight heparin	G	LMWH is not routinely recommended
C	LMHW for 6 weeks after delivery	H	LMWH for 7 days after delivery
D	Mobilization and avoidance of dehydration	I	Graduated compression stocking
E	Thromboprophylaxis with LMWH antenatally and six weeks postpartum	J	Antenatal prophylactic low molecular weight heparin

Instruction: For each question posed below, choose the single **most appropriate thromboprophylaxis** from the A–J list above. The given option may be used once, more than once or not at all.

Question 79	A 32 year old woman is 10 weeks pregnant. She had deep vein thrombosis three years back. Investigation done had shown moderate titer of antiphospholipid antibodies.
Answer 79	
Question 80	A 26 year old second gravida is 6 weeks pregnant. She has moderate titer of antiphospholipid antibody. No other risk factor is present.
Answer 80	

Answers and explanations

Answer 79 (E) Thromboprophylaxis with LMWH antenatally and six weeks postpartum

Women with previous thrombosis and antiphospholipid syndrome should be offered both antenatal and 6 weeks of postpartum thromboprophylaxis.

Pulmonary thromboembolism (PTE) remains the commonest cause of maternal death in the UK. The latest Confidential Enquiry into Maternal and Child Health has highlighted the risk of thromboembolism from the beginning of pregnancy and the need for a full risk assessment at booking.

Answer 80 (H) LMWH for 7 days after delivery

Women with persistent antiphospholipid antibodies with no previous VTE or other risk factors may be managed with close surveillance antenatally. However, LMWH for 7 days postpartum should be considered.

Options for questions 81 – 82

A	Regional analgesia is contraindicated. Alternative analgesia may be offered	F	Stop thromboprophylaxis at least 4 hours before regional anesthesia
B	Stop thromboprophylaxis at least 24 hours before regional anesthesia	G	Stop thromboprophylaxis at least 12 hours before regional anesthesia
C	Should not inject LMWH	H	LMWH should be started eight hours postoperatively
D	Regional analgesia may be administered	I	Dose of heparin should be reduced
E	LMWH should be started four hours postoperatively	J	No need to stop anticoagulants

Instruction: For each question posed below, choose the single most appropriate answer from the A–J list above. The given option may be used once, more than once or not at all.

Question 81	A 27 year old woman has presented in spontaneous labour at 39 weeks of pregnancy. She is contracting 3 in 10 min. On vaginal examination os is 4 cm dilated and 60% effaced. She is requesting regional analgesia. She was receiving thomboprophylaxsis with LMWH. Her last injection was 8 hours ago.
Answer 81	
Question 82	A 26 year old woman has presented in spontaneous labour at 37 weeks of pregnancy. She is contracting 4 in 10 min. On vaginal examination, os is 3 cm dilated and 40% effaced. She is requesting regional analgesia. She had DVT during pregnancy and is receiving therapeutic dose of LMWH. Her last injection was 12 hours ago.
Answer 82	

Answers and explanations

Answer 81 (A) Regional analgesia is contraindicated. Alternative analgesia may be offered

If the woman presents in spontaneous labour within 12 hours of taking a prophylactic, LMWH regional analgesia should be deferred. Alternative analgesia such as opiate-based intravenous or patient-controlled analgesia can be offered.

Answer 82 (A) Regional analgesia is contraindicated. Alternative analgesia may be offered

This woman is on a therapeutic regimen of LMWH, which was injected 12 hours ago. Regional analgesis should not be used for at least 24 hours after the last dose to avoid the risk of epidural haematoma.

Options for questions 83 – 84

A	Start diazepam infusion	F	Call for help
B	Change to phenytoin regimen	G	Give pethidine and phenergan injection
C	Increase dose of magnesium infusion to 3g per hour	H	Increase dose of magnesium infusion to 1.5g per hour
D	Decrease dose of magnesium infusion to 1g per hour	I	Decrease dose of magnesium infusion to 0.5g per hour
E	Stop magnesium sulphate infusion	J	Call anaesthetist

Instruction: For each question posed below, choose the single most appropriate answer from the A–J list above. The given option may be used once, more than once or not at all.

Question 83	A 26 year old primigravida is admitted in A&E with convulsion. Her BP is 160/110 mmHg and three plus proteinuria. Her LFT, U&E is within normal limit. She is on magnesium and labetalol infusion. Magnesium infusion is at the rate of 1 g/hour. She is getting recurrent convulsion.
Answer 83	
Question 84	A 28 year old primigravida is getting convulsion at 32 weeks. Her BP is 150/106 mmHg and two plus proteinuria. She is on magnesium sulphate infusion of 1 g/hour. There is loss of deep tendon reflexes.
Answer 84	

Answers and explanations

Answer 83 (H) Increase dose of magnesium infusion to 1.5g per hour

Magnesium sulphate is the therapy of choice to control seizures. A loading dose of 4g should be given by infusion pump over 5–10 minutes, followed by a further infusion of 1g/hour maintained for 24 hours after the last seizure. Recurrent seizures should be treated with either a further bolus of 2g magnesium sulphate or an increase in the infusion rate to 1.5g or 2.0g per hour. Magnesium sulphate is the therapy of choice and diazepam and phenytoin should no longer be used as first-line drugs.

Answer 84 (E) Stop magnesium sulphate infusion

Patients receiving magnesium sulphate should be monitored carefully for signs and symptoms of magnesium toxicity. Magnesium toxicity manifests initially as loss of patellar reflexes and shortness of breath. Therefore, the patellar reflexes must be checked every 4 hours along with oxygen saturation and the respiratory rate must be monitored. As magnesium sulphate is excreted by the kidney, urine output should be monitored closely and should be at least 30 mL/h. If magnesium toxicity is suspected, a blood test for the magnesium level should be performed. Most practitioners feel comfortable with a level below 9.0 mg/dL. However, patients have been reported to show signs of toxicity below 6.0 mg/dL. Therefore, clinical evaluation of the patient should continue even if the serum magnesium level is below 9.0 mg/dL. Side effects of IV magnesium administration include flushing, chest heaviness, blurred vision and minor headache. While these are not symptoms of toxicity, it may be reasonable to consider lowering the dose or withholding therapy if they become severe. Magnesium sulphate therapy is contraindicated in patients with myasthenia gravis.

Options for questions 85 – 86

A	Hypertension	F	Corneal haziness
B	Hypotension	G	Convulsions
C	Intrauterine growth retardation	H	Bleeding diathesis
D	Vomiting	I	Vesicular eruption
E	Maculopapular eruption	J	Depression

Instruction: For each question posed below, choose the single **most common side effect** from the A–J list above. The given option may be used once, more than once or not at all.

Question 85	A 36 year old woman has had essential hypertension. Her blood pressure was controlled on atenolol. She is now 6 weeks pregnant. She is hesitant to change her medication.
Answer 85	
Question 86	A 26 year old primigravida has developed pre-eclampsia. Methyldopa 500mg TDS was started. Her BP was controlled with it. She has had normal vaginal delivery. The doctor wants to change the medication.
Answer 86	

Answers and explanations

Answer 85 (C) Intrauterine growth retardation

Hypertension in pregnancy is commonly treated by beta-blockers, however, safety of these agents and in particular of atenolol is controversial. Association with IUGR has been suggested. Most drugs have potential adverse effects during pregnancy and the risk involves both the mother and fetus. Therefore, these should be discussed with the mother prior to the start.

Answer 86 (J) Depression

Methyldopa is a centrally-acting antihypertensive drug and is gradually declining in its usage in pregnancy. It inhibits decarboxylation of dopa to dopamine. The mode of action is by reducing the concentrations of dopamine, 5 - hydroxytryptamine and noradrenaline in peripheral tissues and the CNS.

Cautions/contraindications:

- history of depression, active liver disease
- porphyria, phaeochromocytoma
- increases the CNS toxicity of lithium.

Options for questions 87 – 89

A	Fasting blood glucose at 6 weeks postnatal	G	Oral glucose tolerance test 6 weeks postnatal
B	10mmol/l	H	9.4mmol/l
C	3.5-5.9mmol/l	I	HbA$_{1c}$ below 7.6%
D	HbA$_{1c}$ below 6.1%	J	7.8mmol/l
E	HbA$_{1c}$ below 4%	K	8.7mmol/l
F	2.5–4mmol/l	L	Below 2mmol/l

Instruction: For each question posed below, choose the single most appropriate answer from the list above. The given option may be used once, more than once or not at all.

Question 87	A 36 year old second gravida has come for preconception counselling. She has had one miscarriage. She is diabetic since the last 5 years and is on oral hypoglycemic agent. Her glycosylated haemoglobin is 11%. She has been asked to reduce it. At what level should she aim to maintain it?
Answer 87	
Question 88	A 34 year old insulin-dependent diabetic primigravida has attended the antenatal clinic at 6 weeks. Her fasting blood sugar level is within the normal limit but her one hour blood glucose is very high. She has been asked to keep it under control.
Answer 88	
Question 89	A 38 year old Asian woman has attended the antenatal clinic at 12 weeks. She is diabetic and her fasting blood sugar level is 7.6mmol/l. She is not on any hypoglycemic drug. She is enquiring about target fasting blood sugar levels during pregnancy.
Answer 89	

Answers and explanations

Answer 87 (D) HbA$_{1c}$ below 6.1%

Women with diabetes should be counselled to keep their HbA$_{1c}$ below 6.1% if possible. It is likely to decrease the risk of congenital malformations and fetal macrosomia and other complications in the mother and the fetus.

Answer 88 (J) 7.8mmol/l

1-hour postprandial blood glucose should be kept below 7.8mmol/litre during pregnancy, if it is safely achievable.

Answer 89 (C) 3.5–5.9mmol/l

If it is safely achievable, women with diabetes should aim to keep fasting blood glucose between 3.5 and 5.9 mmol/litre.

The following table summarises the 2006 WHO recommendations for the diagnostic criteria for diabetes and intermediate hyperglycaemia.

Diabetes

Fasting plasma glucose or	≥7.0mmol/l (126 mg/dl)
2–h plasma glucose*	≥11.1mmol/l (200 mg/dl)

Impaired Glucose Tolerance (IGT)

Fasting plasma glucose   <7.0mmol/l (126 mg/dl)

2–h plasma glucose*   ≥7.8 and <11.1mmol/l
(140 mg/dl and 200 mg/dl)

Impaired Fasting Glucose (IFG)

Fasting plasma glucose   6.1 to 6.9mmol/l
(110 mg/dl to 125 mg/dl)

2–h plasma glucose (if measured)**   7.8mmol/l
(140 mg/dl)

*Venous plasma glucose 2–h after ingestion of 75g oral glucose load

**If 2–h plasma glucose is not measured, status is uncertain as diabetes or IGT cannot be excluded.

Options for questions 90 – 92

A	Offer random blood sugar for screening	**G**	Offer 2 hour 75 gram oral GTT at 24–28 weeks
B	Offer 2 hour 50 gram GTT at booking and 28 weeks	**H**	Offer 2 hour 50 gram oral GTT at booking
C	Fasting and 2 hour postprandial blood glucose	**I**	Offer 2 hour 50 gram oral GTT at 24–28 weeks
D	Offer 2 hour 75 gram oral GTT at booking	**J**	Offer 2 hour 75 gram oral GTT at 32 weeks
E	Offer fasting plasma glucose for screening	**K**	Offer 2 hour 75 gram oral GTT at 16–18 weeks
F	Offer glucose urine analysis for screening	**L**	Offer 2 hour 75 gram oral GTT at 28 weeks

Instruction: For each question posed below, choose the single most appropriate answer from the A–L list above. The given option may be used once, more than once or not at all.

Question 90	A 30 year old second gravida has come for antenatal care. She had gestational diabetes in her previous pregnancy and delivery was complicated by shoulder dystocia. She is currently 10 weeks pregnant.
Answer 90	
Question 91	A 38 year old third gravida has come for booking. It was noted that her BMI is 34 and her father was diabetic. Her previous two pregnancies were uncomplicated and she had normal deliveries at term.
Answer 91	
Question 92	A 29 year old second gravida has come for her antenatal checkup at 24 weeks. She had gestational diabetes in her previous pregnancy. It was well controlled and she had delivered normally at term. This pregnancy was uncomplicated till date and oral GTT done earlier is normal.
Answer 92	

Answers and explanations

Answer 90 (K) Offer 2 hour 75 gram oral GTT at 16–18 weeks

Gestational diabetes affects 3–10% of pregnancies and is most commonly diagnosed by screening during pregnancy. The specific cause is unknown, however pregnancy hormones believe to increase insulin resistance, resulting in impaired glucose tolerance. It causes macrosomic babies and complications related to it.

Risk factors for developing gestational diabetes:

- a previous gestational diabetes or prediabetes, impaired glucose tolerance, or impaired fasting glycaemia
- a family history revealing a first degree relative with type 2 diabetes
- maternal age (women over 35 years of age)
- ethnic background (African-Americans, Afro-Caribbeans, South Asians)
- body mass index above 30kg/m2
- a previous macrosomic baby weighing 4.5kg or above
- previous poor obstetric history
- a double risk of GDM in smokers
- polycystic ovarian syndrome (relevant evidence remains controversial).

Screening for gestational diabetes using fasting plasma glucose, random blood glucose, glucose challenge test and urinalysis should not be undertaken.

Answer 91 (G) Offer 2 hour 75 gram oral GTT at 24–28 weeks

Answer 92 (L) If the oral GTT done earlier is normal offer 2 hour 75 gram oral GTT at 28 weeks

The 2 hour 75 g oral glucose tolerance test (OGTT) should be used and diagnosis should be made using the criteria defined by the World Health Organisation. Women with a previous history should be offered early OGTT at 16–18 and at 28 weeks (if results are normal) and with any other risk factors at 24–28 weeks.

Options for questions 93 – 95

A	Emergency LSCS	H	Episiotomy
B	Instrumental delivery	I	Fundal pressure
C	Elective caesarean section should be considered	J	Extraction of baby under general anesthesia
D	Elective caesarean section is not recommended	K	Lovset maneuver
E	Induction of labour	L	McRoberts' maneuver
F	Mc william maneuver	M	Knee-chest position
G	Induction of labour is not recommended	N	Rubin maneuver

Instruction: For each question posed below, choose the single most appropriate answer from the A–N list above. The given option may be used once, more than once or not at all.

Question 93	USG of a 32 year old second gravida at 38 weeks woman suspects fetal macrosomia (estimated fetal weight over 4.5kg). She is not diabetic. She requests an elective caesarean section.
Answer 93	
Question 94	Large for date fetus is suspected during the ANC checkup of 30 year old diabetic woman. Fetal macrosomia (estimated fetal weight over 4.5kg) is confirmed by USG scan. She wants to discuss the mode of delivery.
Answer 94	
Question 95	A 34 year old third gravida is about to deliver at 42 weeks of gestation. The midwife notices that during delivery, the head remained tightly applied to the vulva and was even retracting with contraction. She calls for help.
Answer 95	

Answers and explanations

Answer 93 (D) Elective caesarean section is not recommended

The prenatal diagnosis of macrosomia remains imprecise. Pre-pregnancy and antepartum risk factors and ultrasound have poor predictive value. Induction of labour and prophylactic caesarean delivery has not been shown to alter the incidence of shoulder dystocia among nondiabetic patients.

Caesarean section and the induction of labour are associated with an increased risk of operative morbidity and mortality, with added cost implications.

The risk of shoulder dystocia rises from 1.4% for all vaginal deliveries to 9.2–24% for birth weights of more than 4,500 g. Unfortunately, 50% of all cases of shoulder dystocia occur at birth weights of less than 4,000 gm.

Brachial plexus injury occurs in 1:1,000 births and permanent damage in 1:10,000 deliveries (12% of all), leading to litigation 1:45,000 deliveries.

Answer 94 (C) Elective caesarean section should be considered

Fetal macrosomia associated with diabetes, indicates poor maternal glucose control, and these infants are at risk of stillbirth and shoulder dystocia. Planned caesarean section should be considered for women with diabetes and suspected fetal macrosomia to reduce the potential morbidity.

Answer 95 (L) McRoberts' maneuver

The McRoberts' maneuvre involves hyperflexion and abduction of the maternal hips, positioning the maternal thighs tightly to her abdomen. This widens the pelvis, and flattens the spine in the lower back. It is also associated with an increase in uterine pressure and amplitude of contractions.

The McRoberts' maneuver is the single most effective intervention with reported success rates as high as 90%.

Options for questions 96 – 97

A	LFT should be done after 10 days	**F**	LFT to be measured in each trimester
B	LFT should be done after 7 days	**G**	LFT to be measured monthly
C	LFT to be measured weekly	**H**	LFT should be done after 6 weeks
D	LFT to be measured biweekly	**I**	LFT should be done after 6 months
E	LFT to be measured fortnightly	**J**	LFT should be done after 4 weeks

Instruction: For each question posed below, choose the single most appropriate answer from the A–J list above. The given option may be used once, more than once or not at all.

Question 96	A 26 year old primigravida with obstetric cholestasis has been delivered by LSCS at 38 weeks of gestation. Labour was induced with prostin. CS was done for secondary arrest of cervical dilatation. Her ALT was 200 IU/ml due to obstetric cholestasis.
Answer 96	
Question 97	A 28 year old primigravida is complaining of pruritis typically of the palm and sole at night. She is 32 weeks pregnant. Other causes of pruritis have been excluded. Her LFT is mildly deranged. Obstetric cholestasis is diagnosed.
Answer 97	

Answers and explanations

Answer 96 (A) LFT should be done after 10 days

Obstetric cholestasis is an uncommon complication of pregnancy which causes a build-up of bile acids in the bloodstream. The main symptom is persistent itching that occurs most commonly in the third trimester of pregnancy. There is possibly a small increased risk of complications of pregnancy, but the evidence for this is not conclusive.

It is also the second most common cause of jaundice in pregnancy. Other problems with the liver should be considered such as pre-eclampsia, HELLP syndrome, and acute fatty liver of pregnancy. Furthermore, other causes of hepatitis and certain medications should also be considered.

Answer 97 (C) LFT to be measured weekly

Pruritis of palms and soles with raised ALT level is diagnostic of intrahepatic cholestasis (however, LFTs are not always elevated). The serum bile acid blood test is a quantitative measurement of bile salts. The results of this test often take longer to return, but the test is more specific.

Transaminases range from just above the upper limit of normal to several hundreds. Once obstetric cholestasis is diagnosed, LFTs should be measured weekly. Postnatal LFTs should be deferred for at least 10 days.

Options for questions 98 – 99

A	Dexamethasone	G	Activated charcoal
B	Ursodeoxycholic acid	H	Vitamin K 10mg daily orally
C	Vitamin K 10mg daily parentally	I	Vitamin K 20mg daily orally
D	Cholestyramine	J	S-Adenosyl methionine
E	Chlopheniramine	K	Guar gum
F	Prednisolone	L	Induce labour

Instruction: For each question posed below, choose the single most appropriate answer from the A–L list above. The given option may be used once, more than once or not at all.

Question 98	A 30 year old second gravida is complaining of pruritis, which is more severe at night. She is 32 weeks pregnant. All investigations including LFT, USG is normal. She is distressed due to the pruritis.
Answer 98	
Question 99	A 26 year old primigravida has been diagnosed with obstetric choestasis. She is 34 weeks pregnant. All investigations including LFT, USG are normal. She is complaining of frank steatorrhoea.
Answer 99	

Answers and explanations

Answer 98 (B) Ursodeoxycholic acid

This is a naturally occurring bile acid and is used as a medication. It is not licensed for pregnant women, but has often been prescribed to help to reduce the bile acid level in the bloodstream. This may then ease symptoms and may perhaps reduce any possible increased risk of pregnancy complications.

However, the evidence to support the use of this drug is not strong. Current national guidelines on obstetric cholestasis states that there is insufficient data to support the widespread use of ursodeoxycholic acid (UDCA) outside of clinical trials.

Dexamethasone should not be first-line therapy for obstetric cholestasis, nor should it be used outside of an RCT without a thorough consultation with the woman.

Answer 99 (H) Vitamin K 10mg daily orally

Vitamin K is essential for the blood clotting mechanism to work. Sometimes the level is reduced in people with liver and bile problems and therefore supplements are often advised.

Options for questions 100 – 102

A	Ebstein's anomaly	G	Arnold-Chiari malformation
B	Primary pulmonary hypertension	H	Maternal agranulocytosis
C	Cleft lip and palate	I	Neural tube defect
D	Fetal agranulocytosis	J	Gestational diabetes

| E | Floppy baby syndrome | K | High blood pressure |
| F | Duodenal atresia | L | Difficult to withdraw |

Instruction: For each question posed below, choose the single **most appropriate adverse effects** from the list above. The given option may be used once, more than once or not at all.

Question 100	A 29 year old woman was diagnosed to have bipolar disorder. She has been on lithium for the last three years. She is planning pregnancy, visited the doctor for preconception counselling and has been advised to gradually stop lithium.
Answer 100	
Question 101	A 30 year old woman is taking clozapine. She has visited her GP as her urine pregnancy test is positive. She is advised to stop it gradually and another antipsychotic is prescribed for her.
Answer 101	
Question 102	A 25 year old woman has attended the antenatal clinic at 5 weeks. She had seziures 1 year ago and since then she has been on sodium valporate. She is referred to a physician for the change of medication.
Answer 102	

Answers and explanations

Answer 100 (A) Ebstein's anomaly

Lithium increases congenital heart defects to around 60 in 1000 (compared with 8 in 1000 in the general population). It has been seen that Ebstein's anomaly increases by 10 times. Lithium should be avoided in pregnancy especially in the first trimester and during breastfeeding as it is secreted in breast milk in high levels.

Answer 101 (D) Fetal agranulocytosis

Clozapine should not be used during pregnancy or lactation as there is a theoretical risk of agranulocytosis in the fetus. If a woman was found to be pregnant on clozapine then she should be switched onto a different drug.

Answer 102 (I) Neural tube defect

Valporate increases the risk of neural tube defects e.g. spina bifida and anencephaly. It goes up from around 6 in 10,000 pregnancies in the general population to around 100 to 200 in 10,000 in pregnant women on valporate. It should be cautiously prescribed in young women as many pregnancies are not confirmed until after the 28th day (when the neural tube closes).

(Reference – RCOG nos. 37A & B, 10A, 42, 43. NICE guidelines CG 45 2007, CG 63 2007)

EMQs on Antenatal, Intrapartum and Postpartum Problems

Options for questions 103 – 104

A	Uterine artery Doppler	**F**	MRI
B	Assessment of venous blood flow in fetus	**G**	Fetal echo cadiography
C	Assessment of liquor volume	**H**	Umbilical artery Doppler
D	USG-anomaly scan	**I**	USG-biophysical profile
E	CT scan	**J**	CTG

Instruction: For each question posed below, choose the single most appropriate answer from the A–J list above. The given option may be used once, more than once or not at all.

Question 103	A 18 year old primigravida had spontaneous pregnancy while using contraceptive pills. Her routine anomaly scan was normal. Her pregnancy was progressing well until 30 weeks of gestation when she was found to have small for gestational age fetus. USG scan performed suggested AC and EFW less than 10th centile.
Answer 103	
Question 104	A 24 year old primigravida has recently come to the UK at 28 weeks of gestation based on her last menstrual period. She had her first antenatal checkup with her midwife and found to have small for gestational age fetus. There is no record of her care and she does not speak English very well.
Answer 104	

Answers and explanations

Answer 103 (H) Umbilical artery Doppler

In most cases of IUGR, especially those due to primary placental insufficiency, the fetal abdomen is small, but the head and extremities are normal or near normal. This finding is known as the head-sparing effect or asymmetrical IUGR. In cases of severe, early-onset IUGR (those due to chromosomal anomalies), the fetus tends to be symmetrically smaller.

The use of Doppler ultrasonography to measure umbilical artery waveforms should be considered as a part of fetal evaluation once IUGR is suspected or diagnosed. If the Resistance Index increases to a value above the upper range of normal, this identifies a fetus at risk.

Absent blood flow during diastole is a more serious form than decreased blood flow during diastole. Fetuses with this type of finding should be monitored closely in a hospital setting.

Reverse blood flow during diastole occurs when the resistance in the placenta increases further. Recent studies have found that surveillance of high-risk fetuses with umbilical artery Doppler ultrasound results in a marked decrease in fetal death and morbidity when compared to traditional surveillance (non-stress test).

Answer 104 (D) USG-anomaly scan

Up to 19% of fetuses with an AC and EFW less than the fifth centile may have chromosomal defects. Therefore, when a fetus is diagnosed to be small for dates, the risk of chromosomal defects should be assessed. The risk of chromosomal defect is higher when growth restriction is associated with other structural abnormalities, normal liquor volume or a normal uterine or umbilical artery Doppler.

All growth-restricted fetuses should have an ultrasound anatomical survey as a minimum to exclude any structural anomaly. It may also be appropriate to offer karyotyping if there is any doubt.

Options for questions 105 – 108

A	Repeat uterine artery Doppler fortnightly	I	Assessment of liquor volume
B	Assessment of venous blood flow in fetus	J	Delay delivery till 37 weeks
C	Repeat umbilical artery Doppler weekly	K	Repeat umbilical artery Doppler biweekly
D	Immediate delivery	L	Biophysical profile
E	USG-biophysical profile	M	Administration of steroids
F	CTG daily	N	Amniocentesis
G	Steroid and tocolysis	O	Admit in hospital
H	Repeat umbilical artery Doppler fortnightly	P	MCA Doppler

Instruction: For each question posed below, choose the single most appropriate answer from the A–P list above. The given option may be used once, more than once or not at all.

Question 105	A 30 year old multigravida in her third pregnancy was booked at 11 weeks. She had two previous small babies. First trimester screening has suggested low risk for chromosomal anomaly. Her 20 week's anomaly scan was also normal. Ultrasound scan performed showed AC and EFW less than 10th centile at 30 weeks of gestation. Umbilical artery doppler performed is normal.
Answer 105	
Question 106	A 32 year old primigravida is seen in the antenatal clinic at 32 weeks of gestation. Her fundal height suggested small for dates, therefore an ultrasound scan was performed. The AC and EFW were noted to be less than 10th centile. Umbilical artery Doppler suggested high pulsality index but end diastolic flow is present. Other surveillance tests are normal. Repeat Doppler was within normal range.
Answer 106	
Question 107	A 26 year old primigravida had an uneventful pregnancy until 32 weeks of gestation when the fundal height was noted to be 4 cm less than expected. Her anomaly scan was normal. Ultrasound scan performed showed AC and EFW less than 10th centile. Umbilical artery Doppler showed reversed end diastolic flow. Other surveillance tests are normal.
Answer 107	
Question 108	A 28 year old primigravida was found to have small for dates at 32 weeks of gestation and showed AC and EFW less than 10th centile. Her anomaly scan was normal. Umbilical artery Doppler suggested reversed end diastolic flow. Doppler of ductus venous performed is also abnormal.
Answer 108	

Answers and explanations

Answer 105 (H) Repeat umbilical artery Doppler fortnightly

SGA fetuses should be monitored with umbilical artery Doppler. The evidence suggests that monitoring with twice-weekly umbilical artery Doppler compared with fortnightly monitoring result in earlier delivery and increased incidence of the induction of labour. There is no difference in neonatal morbidity or mortality. This suggests the frequency of monitoring in SGA fetuses with normal Doppler should be repeated every fortnight.

Answer 106 (J) Delay delivery till 37 weeks

When end diastolic flow is present (PED), delivery should be delayed until at least 37 weeks, provided other surveillance findings are normal. This will avoid prematurity and complications associated with it. In the absence of effective fetal therapies, timing of delivery becomes the critical issue. The risk of intrauterine compromise has to be weighed against the potential risks from iatrogenic premature delivery (before 32–34 weeks' gestation).

Arterial and venous Doppler parameters, biophysical variables and CTG are used for the fetal surveillance. Studies suggest that the diagnosis of IUGR is associated with an increased iatrogenic prematurity.

Answer 107 (M) Administration of steroids

When end diastolic flow is absent or reversed then the woman should be offered admission for close surveillance including CTG monitoring. Administration of steroids should be considered in case premature delivery is expedited.

Answer 108 (D) Immediate delivery

When end diastolic flow is absent or reversed, admission for close surveillance and administration of steroids is required. If other surveillance results (biophysical profile, venous Doppler) are abnormal, delivery is indicated. If gestation is over 34 weeks, even if other results are normal, delivery may be considered.

Options for questions 109 – 111

A	Instrumental delivery	G	Vaginal delivery
B	Urgent caesarean section	H	Speculum examination
C	Wrap saline soaked swab around the cord	I	Elevate the presenting part manually
D	Offer immediate admission	J	Offer admission at 36 weeks of gestation
E	Offer admission	K	Tocolysis
F	Offer admission to hospital after 37+6 weeks of gestation	L	Manual replacement of the prolapsed cord above the presenting part

Instruction: For each question posed below, choose the single most **appropriate initial management for appropriate management** from the A–L list above. The given option may be used once, more than once or not at all.

Question 109	A 30 year old multigravida attends antenatal clinic at 34 weeks of pregnancy. On abdominal examination, transverse lie of fetus is suspected. USG scan confirmed transverse lie. Her BP is 136/84 mmHg. She is very anxious.
Answer 109	
Question 110	A 36 year old primigravida is admitted with labour pains. On examination cervix is 3 cm dilated, 90% effaced, bag of membrane is bulging and presenting part is cephalic which is high. CTG is normal. After an hour the midwife calls for help as she notices abnormalities in CTG tracing just after rupture of membrane. Cord is seen coming through the vagina.
Answer 110	
Question 111	A 36 year old primigravida is admitted with labour pains. Two hours later she developed CTG abnormalities. Examination confirmed cord prolapse. She is contracting 4 in 10. On vaginal examination cervix is 4 cm dilated, 80% effaced, cord is in the vagina, and presentation is vertex. The abnormalities in CTG tracing persists even after mechanical methods have taken place and delivery is likely to be delayed.
Answer 111	

Answers and explanations

Answer 109 (F) Offer admission to hospital after 37+6 weeks of gestation

Elective hospital admission after 37+6 weeks of gestation should be discussed with transverse, oblique or unstable lie. Cord prolapse occurring in hospital have better outcomes than those occurring outside the hospital setting. Rapid assessment once labour starts or after spontaneous rupture of membranes is advised to these women.

Answer 110 (I) Elevate the presenting part manually

Presenting part should be pushed away from the pelvis to avoid cord compression. This can be done manually (presenting part can be pushed upwards vaginally with the examining fingers). Once the presenting part is above the pelvic brim, continuous suprapubic pressure in an upwards direction should be used. Filling the urinary bladder also helps in disengaging presenting part to avoid cord compression.

The mother adopting the knee-chest position or head-down tilt (preferably in left-lateral position) can further reduce cord compression.

Answer 111 (K) Tocolysis

Tocolysis can be considered with terbutaline 0.25mg subcutaneus to reduce contractions. If there are persistent fetal heart rate trace abnormalities despite attempts to prevent cord compression and there is a delay in achieving delivery, tocolysis should be given.

Options for questions 112 – 114

A	At 34 weeks	H	At 36–37 weeks
B	Every 2–3 weeks from 16 weeks	I	Every 2–3 weeks from 10 weeks
C	At 31 weeks	J	At 33 weeks
D	At 32 weeks	K	At 39 weeks
E	Weekly from 20 weeks	L	At 38 weeks
F	Weekly from 16 weeks	M	At 35 weeks
G	Every 2–3 weeks from 24 weeks	N	Every 4 weeks from 24 weeks

Instruction: For each question posed below, choose the single most appropriate answer from the A–N list above. The given option may be used once, more than once or not at all.

Question 112	A 36 year old conceived after in-vitro fertilization. USG scan done at 6 weeks shows monochorionic diamniotic pregnancy. She has had an uncomplicated pregnancy so far. She has come for a checkup at 32 weeks and wants to discuss the timing of the induction of pregnancy.
Answer 112	
Question 113	USG scan done at 9 weeks shows monochorionic monoamniotic twin pregnancy. She is a 40 year old primigravida. She has attended the antenatal clinic at 28 weeks. The plan of delivery is being discussed.
Answer 113	
Question 114	A 36 year old third gravida is diagnosed to have monochorionic twin pregnancy by USG scan at 10 weeks. It is a spontaneous conception. Her previous pregnancies were uncomplicated and had delivered normally. Her antenatal follow-up is being planned.
Answer 114	

Answers and explanations

Answer 112 (H) At 36–37 weeks

Normal incidence of twins is 1 in 80–90 pregnancies (approximately 1/3 are monozygotic) and of triplets, 1 in 8100 pregnancies. However, use of in-vitro fertilisation (IVF) and ovulation induction techniques has greatly increased the incidence of multiple pregnancies.

There is a higher risk of unexplained fetal demise despite intensive fetal surveillance. Therefore delivery should be planned for 36-37 weeks of gestation, for uncomplicated MCDC pregnancies (without TTTS or fetal growth restriction). However, this is not based on any randomized study and controversy continues.

Answer 113 (D) At 32 weeks

Monochorionic (MC) and dichorionic (DC) twin pregnancies share increased risks of preterm birth, fetal growth restriction, pre-eclampsia and postpartum haemorrhage. The particular challenges of monochorionic pregnancies arise from the vascular placental anastomoses that are almost universal and connect the umbilical circulations of both twins. TTTS complicates 10–15% of MC pregnancies.

In addition, monochorionic, monoamniotic pregnancies (1% of twin pregnancies) carry a very high risk of cord entanglement. Therefore many clinicians recommend delivery by caesarean section at 32 weeks after corticosteroids to avoid cord entanglement.

Answer 114 (B) Every 2–3 weeks from 16 weeks

Fetal ultrasound assessment should take place every 2–3 weeks in uncomplicated monochorionic pregnancies from 16 weeks. Ultrasound examinations between 16 and 24 weeks focus primarily on the detection of TTTS.

After 24 weeks, when first presentation of TTTS is uncommon, the main purpose is to detect fetal growth restriction, which may be concordant or discordant.

Options for questions 115 – 117

A	Integrated test (nuchal translucency, beta human chorionic gonadotropin, pregnancy-associated plasma protein-A serum inhibin, alpha-fetoprotein, estriol) at 20 weeks	**F**	Integrated test (nuchal translucency, beta human chorionic gonadotropin, pregnancy-associated plasma protein-A, serum inhibin, alpha-fetoprotein, estriol) at 12 weeks
B	Quadruple test (beta human chorionic gonadotropin, serum inhibin, alpha-fetoprotein, and estriol) at 16 weeks	**G**	Quadruple test (beta human chorionic gonadotropin, serum inhibin, alpha-fetoprotein, estriol) at 24 weeks
C	No need for the test as she is not a high risk. She should have routine anomaly scan at 21 weeks which will exclude any anomaly	**H**	Combined test (nuchal translucency, beta human chorionic gonadotropin, pregnancy-associated plasma protein-A) at 15 weeks
D	Combined test (nuchal translucency, beta human chorionic gonadotropin, pregnancy-associated plasma protein-A) at 11 weeks	**I**	Combined test (nuchal translucency, beta human chorionic gonadotropin, pregnancy-associated plasma protein-A) at 18 weeks
E	Quadruple test (beta human chorionic gonadotropin, serum inhibin, alpha fetoprotein, estriol) at 14 weeks	**J**	Soft tissue marker for Down's syndrome can be looked for at anomaly scan

Instruction: For each question posed below, choose the single most appropriate answer from the A–J list above. The given option may be used once, more than once or not at all.

Question 115	A 26 year old woman is 6 weeks pregnant. This is her first pregnancy. Her elder sister had baby at the age of 38 years. Baby was diagnosed to have Down's syndrome after birth. She would like to be screened as early as possible.
Answer 115	
Question 116	A 36 year old second gravida has come for booking at 14 weeks of gestation. Her first baby was born by LSCS 2 years ago. The baby is doing well. Her antenatal plan is being discussed. She would like to know at what gestational age she will be screened for Down's syndrome. Her anomaly scan is booked at 19 weeks.
Answer 116	
Question 117	A 34 year old second gravida with BMI 34 is booked for a scan for first trimester screening (Down's syndrome) at 12 weeks 5 days. During the scan it was difficult to measure nuchal translucency. She is given another appointment.
Answer 117	

Answers and explanations

Answer 115 (D) Combined test (nuchal translucency, beta human chorionic gonadotropin, pregnancy associated plasma protein-A) at 11 weeks

The combined test should be offered to screen for Down's syndrome between 11 completed weeks and 13 weeks 6 days. The cut-off level for screen positive in first trimester screening is 1:150 at term.

Answer 116 (B) Quadruple test (beta human chorionic gonadotropin, serum inhibin, alpha-fetoprotein, estriol) at 16 weeks

For women who book later in pregnancy (between 15 weeks and 20 completed weeks), the quadruple test should be offered. Approximately 15% of the population book late in pregnancy. The cut-off level for screen positive in second trimester screening is 1:200 at term.

Answer 117 (B) Quadruple test (beta human chorionic gonadotropin, serum inhibin, alpha-fetoprotein, estriol) at 16 weeks

Sometimes, it is not possible to measure NT. This is either due to fetal position or raised BMI. In such cases serum screening can be offered between 15 weeks and 20 completed weeks. Down's syndrome screening using soft markers at anomaly scan is not recommended.

Screening tests for Down's syndrome

Screen	Time performed	Detection rate	False +ve rate	Description
Quad Test	15 to 20 weeks	81%	5%	This test measures the maternal serum alpha feto-protein, estriol, human chorionic gonadotropin, and inhibin
Combined Test	11 to 13+ [6] weeks	85%	5%	NT/ free beta hCG and / PAPP A screen
Integrated Test	11 to 13+[6] & 15 to 20 weeks	95%	5%	The integrated test uses measurements from both the 1st trimester combined and the 2nd trimester quad test to yield a more accurate screening result

Options for questions 118 – 119

A	Crown-rump length	F	Humerus length
B	Biparietal diameter	G	Doppler imaging
C	Head circumference	H	Femur length
D	Head circumference/ Abdominal circumference ratio	I	Femur length / Abdominal circumference ratio
E	Biparietal diameter/ Abdominal circumference) ratio	J	Crown-rump length/ Abdominal circumference ratio

Instruction: For each question posed below, choose the single **most appropriate parameter to know gestational age** from the A–J list above. The given option may be used once, more than once or not at all.

Question 118	A 35 year old primigravida is undergoing USG scan for gestational age. Her previous cycles were irregular, therefore she was prescribed an oral contraceptive pill. She stopped this three months ago. Her last menstrual period was about two months ago.
Answer 118	
Question 119	A 34 year old multigravida has conceived during lactational amenorrhoea. On examination the uterus is not palpable abdominally. USG scan shows crown-rump length of 90mm and cardiac activity is present.
Answer 119	

Answers and explanations

Answer 118 (A) Crown-rump length

The 3 basic methods used to help estimate gestational age (GA) are menstrual history, clinical examination and ultrasonography. The first 2 are subject to considerable error and should only be used when ultrasonography facilities are not available.

Ultrasound examination of the fetus provides the most precise assessment of gestational age in the first trimester. Significant reduction in post-term induction occurs when gestational age is established by USG. There is excellent correlation between GA and CRL till 12 weeks.

Menstrual age:

- overestimates the gestational age
- 10–45% do not provide correct information
- 18% with certain dates have significant difference with USG age.

Answer 119 (C) Head circumference

Fetal biometry in the second trimester can yield acceptably accurate estimates of gestational age from 12 to approximately 22 weeks. Recent work has shown that the accuracy of ultrasonographic biometry at 12–14 weeks' gestation is at least as good as biometry performed after 14 weeks.

The best parameters are the biparietal diameter (BPD) and the head circumference (HC), which are linearly related to gestational age. If the crown–rump length is above 84 mm, the gestational age should be estimated using head circumference.

Options for questions 120 – 122

A	Before 10 weeks	G	At 30 weeks
B	11–13 completed weeks	H	Before 16 completed weeks
C	At 8 weeks	I	Before 26 weeks
D	15 weeks onwards	J	At any gestation
E	At 9 weeks	K	Around 10–18 weeks
F	20 weeks onwards	L	After 22 weeks

Instruction: For each question posed below, choose the single **most appropriate timing for performing these procedures** from the A–L list above. The given option may be used once, more than once or not at all.

Question 120	A 40 year old woman conceived after IVF. First trimester screening has suggested the risk of Down's syndrome is 1:150. She is very anxious and currently 14 weeks pregnant. She is requesting amniocentesis and wants to know when it can be done.
Answer 120	
Question 121	A primigravida has family history of Tay sachs disease and has been requesting CVS as soon as possible. She is seven weeks pregnant and wants to know how soon this can be done.
Answer 121	
Question 122	A second gravida conceived twins spontaneously. She is currently 20 weeks pregnant. Ultrasound scan for fetal anatomy performed had shown discrepancy in fetal growth and oligohydramnios in one of the twins. Most likely diagnosis is TTTS. A further repeat scan has been advised in one week. She wants to know what the treatment is and until what gestation laser treatment for TTTS can be performed.
Answer 122	

Answers and explanations

Answer 120 (D) 15 weeks onwards

Amniocentesis usually is done in the second trimester between 15 and 20 weeks of pregnancy. Early amniocentesis before 15 weeks is no longer recommended because it poses a higher risk of miscarriage and other complications.

Serious complications from second trimester amniocentesis are uncommon. However, the procedure does pose a small risk of miscarriage (1 in 100). Other complications, such as uterine infections are rare, occurring in less than 1 in 1,000 cases. It may increase the risk of foot deformity (talipes) and respiratory morbidity.

Answer 121 (B) 11–13 completed weeks

CVS carried out before 10 weeks of pregnancy was found to be associated with limb defects. However, other studies suggest that it may not be connected to the procedure. Nevertheless most units only carry out CVS after 10 weeks because of the possible risk and it is done at 11–13 completed weeks.

Answer 122 (I) Before 26 weeks

Laser treatment aims to destroy the abnormal blood vessels in the placenta that are responsible for the poor blood circulation between the two twins.

A telescope is passed through the uterus and into the recipient twin's amniotic sac. A laser beam is then passed through the scope to break the abnormal anastomosis of blood vessels. This laser treatment often helps to normalise blood flow and sometimes works to completely eliminate the TTTS.

Options for questions 123 – 125

A	Uncertainty in the safety and efficacy of planned VBAC	F	VBAC may be considered after consultant assessment
B	Refer to tertiary care	G	Blood transfusion
C	VBAC is contraindicated	H	VBAC is highly successful
D	Elective caesarean section is contraindicated	I	Offer general anaesthesia
E	Epidural anaesthesia may be offered	J	Epidural is contraindicated

Instruction: For each question posed below, choose the single most appropriate answer from the A–J list above. The given option may be used once, more than once or not at all.

Question 123	A 30 year old woman attended antenatal clinic at 34 weeks and wants to discuss the mode of delivery. She had a hysterotomy with a low vertical incision at 22 weeks' gestation two years ago for premature rupture of membranes and chorioamnionitis. She is requesting vaginal birth.
Answer 123	
Question 124	A multigravida in her 5th pregnancy has had previous two LSCS for breech presentations. She has also had two normal deliveries in between of babies weighing 3.5kg approximately. She is adamant for vaginal delivery.
Answer 124	
Question 125	A 26 year old woman has had an uneventful pregnancy. She is not sure about pain relief in labour. While in the first stage of labour she requested gas and air and pethidine, but she is not sure whether they will be effective. She had previous LSCS for breech presentation 3 years ago.
Answer 125	

Answers and explanations

Answer 123 (C) VBAC is contraindicated

Women with a prior history of hysterotomy or classical caesarean section are recommended to deliver by elective CS. The risk of rupture is 2% with prior low vertical incision in the uterus and 2–9% with the classical caesarean section. With prior T and J incision the risk of rupture is almost 2%, therefore an elective caesarean section should be recommended after discussion with the woman.

Answer 124 (F) VBAC may be considered after consultant assessment

VBAC after 2 previous CSs is safe if proper patient selection is carried out and a meticulously high standard of obstetric care is provided. Proper discussion and informed consent should be taken prior to delivery by a consultant obstetrician regarding all complications, including slight increased risk of scar rupture. She should be fully informed regarding increased uterine dehiscence with more than one previous caesarean section (which is slightly higher than with one previous caesarean).

Answer 125 (E) Epidural anaesthesia may be offered

The latest evidence shows that the use of epidurals do not increase the risk for rupture of caesarean scars in the women with VBAC. It does not mask the pain or tenderness of impending uterine rupture. Therefore, epidural anaesthesia is not contraindicated in planned VBAC.

Options for questions 126 – 128

A	Approximately 40%	G	50-60%
B	20%	H	12%
C	72–76%	I	63–70%
D	19%	J	47%
E	87-90%	K	96%
F	80%	L	19%

Instruction: For each question posed below, choose the single most appropriate answer from the A–L list above. The given option may be used once, more than once or not at all.

Question 126	A 27 year old second gravida has come to you at 20 weeks of gestation. She has had a previous caesarean section for suspicious CTG in the first stage of labour two years ago. She wants to discuss the mode of delivery and is asking about the overall success rate of planned VBAC.
Answer 126	
Question 127	A 35 year old in her third pregnancy has attended antenatal clinic at 28 weeks. She had a first baby delivered by LSCS, second was a vaginal birth. She wants to know about the success of vaginal delivery in the current pregnancy.
Answer 127	
Question 128	A 36 year old second gravida has a BMI of 30. She has had a spontaneous uneventful pregnancy so far. She is being offered induction at 41 weeks with favourable cervix. Her first baby was delivered by LSCS for cervical dystocia. She is anxious to know about the success of induction of labour this time.
Answer 128	

Answers and explanations

Answer 126 (C) 72–76%

Women considering their options for vaginal birth after a single previous caesarean section should be informed that the chances of successful planned VBAC are 72–76%. The chance of having a vaginal birth is almost 40–50%, even in women who are not considered suitable.

Success of a VBAC depends on the following factors:

1. Maternal Age
2. Body Mass Index
3. Ethnicity
4. Prior Vaginal Delivery
5. Previous VBAC
6. Potentially recurrent indication for caesarean.

Expectant mothers who are planning a VBAC should be encouraged to do their own research, find out what options they have and learn more about VBAC.

Answer 127 (E) 87–90%

Previous vaginal birth, particularly previous VBAC, is the single best predictor for successful VBAC. It is associated with a success rate of approximately 87–90%.

There is no single factor that can predict successful vaginal birth. However, having a previous vaginal birth, either before or after previous caesarean section, is very strongly associated with VBAC success.

Answer 128 (A) Approximately 40%

Risk factors for unsuccessful VBAC are as mentioned above are induced labour, no previous vaginal birth, and body mass index greater than 30 and previous caesarean section for dystocia.

These factors reduce the success rate of less than 50%.

Options for questions 129 – 131

A	16 weeks	F	10 weeks
B	By posterior midline episiotomy with epidural	G	By mediolateral episiotomy with epidural
C	20 weeks	H	26 weeks
D	Before conception	I	By posterior midline episiotomy
E	By anterior midline episiotomy with epidural or local analgesia	J	By anterior midline episiotomy

Instruction: For each question posed below, choose the single **most appropriate time of defibulation** from the A–J list above. The given option may be used once, more than once or not at all.

Question 129	A 25 year old Somalian woman is planning pregnancy. She has recently arrived in the UK. She has fear of childbirth. On sensitive enquiry and examination it is found that she has type 2 genital mutilation.
Answer 129	
Question 130	A 36 year old primigravida has attended the antenatal clinic at 8 weeks. Sensitive discussion built-up her confidence and she shared her experience of infibulation. She is found to have type three genital mutilation. After appropriate counselling, she is willing for defibulation.
Answer 130	
Question 131	A 34 year old primigravida is admitted in the labour ward with labour pains at 39 weeks. She has had an uncomplicated pregnancy so far. The midwife has called the doctor as she notices type 2 genital mutilation.
Answer 131	

Answers and explanations

Answer 129 (D) Before conception

Women who have had female genital mutilation are significantly more likely to experience difficulties during childbirth. Complications include the need to have a caesarean section, severe postpartum haemorrhage and prolonged hospitalisation following the birth.

Female genital mutilation (FGM) comprises all procedures that involve partial or total removal of the external female genitalia. This also includes other injury to the female genital organs for non-medical reasons.

The degree of complications is increased according to the extent and severity of the procedure. In order to prevent complication during childbirth, women should be recommended to undergo defibulation before conception, especially if difficult surgery is anticipated.

Answer 130 (C) 20 weeks

Antenatal surgical correction should ideally be performed around 20 weeks of gestation to reduce the risk of miscarriage and allow time for healing before the childbirth.

Answer 131 (E) By anterior midline episiotomy with epidural or local analgesia

If there is a problem with vaginal assessment in the case of tight introitus, the scar can be opened along the midline. The incision should be made at the height of a contraction, and usually after the administration of a local anaesthetic. There is a little bleeding from the relatively avascular scar tissue, and suturing of the cut edges can be delayed until after delivery.

Options for questions 132 – 133

A	Mifepristone 200mg three times a day for 2 days	G	Misoprostol 50 micogram every 4 hourly
B	Mifepristone 200mg followed by misoprostol 800 microgram	H	Artificial rupture of membrane followed by oxytocin infusion
C	Mifepristone 200mg followed by misoprostol 50 micogram every 4 hourly	I	Mifepristone 200mg followed by misoprostol 100 micogram every 4 hourly
D	Prostaglandin gel every four hourly	J	Expectant management
E	Hysterotomy	K	Oxytocin infusion
F	Surgical evacuation of uterus	L	LSCS

Instruction: For each question posed below, choose the single most appropriate management from the A–L list above. The given option may be used once, more than once or not at all.

Question 132	A 41 year old primigravida has been referred to the labour ward by her community midwife as she could not hear the fetal heartbeat by sonicaid. On history, the woman had not felt fetal movements for 7 days. She is 30 weeks pregnant. USG done confirmed intrauterine fetal death. She was booked at 10 weeks and the anomaly scan was normal.
Answer 132	
Question 133	A 30 year old second gravida has come to the day assessment unit at 26 weeks. Fetal heart sound was not audible on sonicaid. USG confirmed intrauterine fetal death. She had a caesarean section done for breech presentation 2 years ago. Her first trimester screening was normal and anomaly scan was normal.
Answer 133	

Answers and explanations

Answer 132 (C) Mifepristone 200mg followed by misoprostol 50 microgram every 4 hourly

The addition of mifepristone appeared to reduce the time interval by about 7 hours compared with published regimens not including mifepristone, but there is no other apparent benefit.

A single 200mg dose of mifepristone is appropriate for late IUFD and the dose of misoprostol should be adjusted according to gestational age (100 micrograms 6-hourly before 26 weeks; 25–50 micrograms 4-hourly at 26 weeks or more).

Answer 133 (A) Mifepristone 200mg three times a day for 2 days

However, a discussion of the safety and benefits of induction of labour should be undertaken by a consultant obstetrician. Mifepristone can be used alone to increase the chance of labour significantly within 72 hours (avoiding the use of prostaglandin).

Options for questions 134 – 136

A	Offer induction with oxytocin	F	Offer induction with misoprostol
B	Offer induction of labour or expectant management	G	Offer support to help woman and her partner
C	Offer induction with Foley's catheterization	H	Offer induction with Laminaria tent
D	Offer immediate LSCS	I	Offer induction of labour with mifepristone and vaginal prostaglandins
E	Offer expectant management	J	Offer induction of labour

Instruction: For each question posed below, choose the single **most appropriate initial management** from the A–J list above. The given option may be used once, more than once or not at all.

Question 134	A 38 year old second gravida was admitted for severe PIH at 34 weeks. She is put on labetolol infusion. She is complaining of decreased fetal movement. Fetal heart sound not heard by Doppler. USG confirmed intrauterine fetal death.
Answer 134	
Question 135	USG scan of a 30 year old primigravida confirmed intrauterine fetal death at 32 weeks of pregnancy. On examination she is stable; her pulse is 80/min, BP 120/70 mmhg. Presentation is cephalic and she is not complaining of any leaking or bleeding. She has been given specialist support.
Answer 135	
Question 136	A 26 year old primigravida is complaining of leaking per vaginum for 3 days at 32 weeks. On examination her pulse is 110/min, BP 110/70 mmhg. On examination fetal heart could not be localised with Doppler and USG scan confirmed fetal death. She has been given specialist support.
Answer 136	

Answers and explanations

Answer 134 (G) Offer support to help woman and her partner

In the event of an intrauterine fetal death, healthcare professionals should offer support to women, their partners and/or family to cope with the emotional and physical consequences of the death. This should also include offering information about specialist support.

Answer 135 (B) Offer induction of labour or expectant management

Following an intrauterine fetal death, the choice of the immediate induction of labour or expectant management should be offered. There is no harm in expectant management if membranes are intact and there is no evidence of infection or bleeding. The woman should be given a chance to discuss and decide the timing regarding induction and further management.

Answer 136 (I) Offer induction of labour with mifepristone and vaginal prostaglandins

If there is an evidence of ruptured membranes, infection or bleeding, immediate induction of labour is the preferred management option. Induction of labour with oral mifepristone, followed by vaginal PGE2 or misoprostol, should be considered.

Options for questions 137 – 139

A	FBS should be repeated every 45 minutes	F	FBS should be repeated every 15 minutes
B	Consultant advice should be sought	G	No need to repeat FBS
C	FBS should be repeated every 5 minutes	H	FBS should be repeated in 30 minutes
D	FBS should be repeated in 90 minutes	I	FBS should be repeated in 45 minutes
E	FBS should be repeated in one hour	J	FBS should be repeated in 10 minutes

Instruction: For each question posed below, choose the single most appropriate answer from the A–J list above. The given option may be used once, more than once or not at all.

Question 137	A 32 year old multigravida is in labour at 41 weeks. She had spontaneous rupture of membrane and thick meconium staning of liquor is noticed. Continuous fetal monitoring was done and trace was considered to be pathological. Her FBS showed pH to be 7.26. Fetal heart trace remained the same.
Answer 137	
Question 138	A 26 year old primigravida is in labour at 38 weeks. There was delay in the first stage of labour. Oxytocin drip was started. She has had continuous fetal monitoring. Her tracing showed fetal heart rate baseline to be 109/minute and variable deceleration in over 50% of contraction, occuring for more than 90 minutes. FBS showed pH to be 7.22.
Answer 138	
Question 139	A 36 year old multigravida is in labour at 38 weeks. She is diabetic. Continuous fetal monitoring was done. There were non-reassuring features and it was decided to do FBS. It showed pH to be 7.20. She is 5 cm dilated and 60% effaced. Vertex is at + 1 station.
Answer 139	

Answers and explanations

Answer 137 (E) FBS should be repeated in one hour

Fetal scalp blood sampling is performed in order to assess fetal acidosis, in the presence of a suspicious or pathological CTG. This helps to diagnose level of hypoxia/acidosis in the fetus, to facilitate further obstetric management.

All scalp pH estimations should be interpreted taking into account the previous pH measurement, the rate of progress in labour and the clinical features of the mother and baby. If CTG warrants scalp pH estimations and it is not possible to perform them, then delivery is indicated.

Interpretation of fetal blood sampling result (NICE Guidelines)

FBS Result (pH)	Interpretation	Subsequent Action
>7.25	Normal	Repeat FBS if FHR abnormality persists
7.21 – 7.24	Borderline	Repeat FBS within 30 minutes or consider delivery if rapid fall since last sample
<7.20	Abnormal	Delivery indicated

Interpreting the result

If pH 7.25 or more and base excess/deficit above −10 (e.g. −5)

These are normal non-acidotic values.

If the CTG improves or accelerations develop after the FBS, no further FBS is needed.

If the CTG deteriorates, repeat the FBS in 30 minutes.

If CTG stays the same consider repeating it in no longer than one hour.

If pH between 7.21 and 7.24 and base excess/deficit above −10

This is a borderline result.

Blood sampling should be repeated no more than 30 minutes later if the FHR trace remains suspicious or pathological, or sooner if there are further abnormalities.

If the FHR trace remains unchanged and the FBS result is stable after the second test, a third/further sample may be deferred unless additional abnormalities develop on the trace.

If a third sample needs to be taken consultant on call must be called

If pH 7.20 or less or base excess −10 or below (e.g. −11)

This indicates fetal acidosis.

The baby must be delivered as soon as possible.

All scalp pH estimations should be interpreted taking into account the previous pH results, the rate of progress and the well-being of the mother and baby.

Answer 138 (H) FBS should be repeated in 30 minutes

If the FBS result is borderline sampling should be repeated no more than 30 minutes later if tracing remains same.

Answer 139 (B) Consultant advice should be sought

If FBS result is abnormal, the advice of a consultant or senior obstetrician should be sought.

Options for questions 140 – 142

A	Reduce oxytocin infusion dose	F	Consultant advice should be sought
B	Stop oxytocin infusion	G	Right lateral position
C	Subcutaneous terbutaline 0.25mg	H	Continue with oxytocin infusion
D	Maternal facial oxygen	I	Left lateral position
E	Fetal blood sampling	J	Reassurance

Instruction: For each question posed below, choose the single most appropriate answer from the A–J list above. The given option may be used once, more than once or not at all.

Question 140	A second gravida is in spontaneous labour at 39 weeks. She has had an uncomplicated pregnancy. Continuous fetal monitoring is done on her request. Her baseline is 120/minute, variability is more than 5/minute but she had variable deceleration in over 50% of contraction for 40 minutes.
Answer 140	
Question 141	A 36 year old primigravida is in spontaneous labour at 37 weeks. Oxytocin infusion was started as she had hypotonic uterine contraction. The midwife asks you to review CTG trace. It showed baseline to be 120/minute, variability of more than five beats per minute and no deceleration and acceleration. She is getting 7 uterine contractions in ten minute periods.
Answer 141	
Question 142	A 23 year old primigravida is in spontaneous labour at 40 weeks. The midwife asks you to review CTG trace. It showed baseline to be 100 beats per minute, variability of 2 beats per minute and variable deceleration and no accelerations in a 10 minute period. She is getting eight uterine contractions in ten minute periods.
Answer 142	

Answers and explanations

Answer 140 (I) Left lateral position

If the CTG trace is suspicious, changing position or giving IV fluids should be considered.

Answer 141 (A) Reduce oxytocin infusion dose

If uterine hyperstimulation is evident, the oxytocin infusion dose should be reduced even if FHR trace is normal.

Answer 142 (C) Subcutaneous terbutaline 0.25mg

In cases where uterine hyperstimulation is causing abnormality in CTG (without the use of oxytocin), tocolysis with subcutaneous terbutaline 0.25mg should be considered.

Options for questions 143 – 145

A	Outlet forceps	G	High forceps
B	Ventouse delivery	H	Fetal scalp electode
C	Instrumental delivery is contraindicated	I	Appropriate analgesia
D	Spontaneous delivery	J	Catheterize bladder
E	Classical caesarean section	K	Fundal pressure
F	Low forceps	L	Emergency caesarean section

Instruction: For each question posed below, choose the single most appropriate management answer from the A–L list above. The given option may be used once, more than once or not at all.

Question 143	A primigravida is in labour at 38 weeks of gestation. Midwife has called you as the mother is exhausted and CTG is showing late deceleration. On examination cervix is fully dilated, vertex is at + 1 station and position is occipito anterior.
Answer 143	
Question 144	A second gravida is in spontaneous labour at 33 weeks of gestation. On abdominal examination the head was not palpable. CTG is showing atypical variable deceleration. Vaginal examination done showed fully dilated os, vertex at plus 2 station and direct occipito posterior position.
Answer 144	
Question 145	A 36 year old second gravida has come to the labour ward. CTG is showing typical variable deceleration. On vaginal examination she is 6 cm dilated and 70% effaced and membrane is intact. Head is at +1 station. She had primary herpes simplex infection at 35 weeks.
Answer 145	

Answers and explanations

Answer 143 (B) Ventouse delivery

Since the CTG is abnormal, delivery should be expedited. Vertex is at plus one station with fully dilated cervix and delivery should be conducted by ventouse. This is more popular because of ease of its use and the fact that it less traumatic to the mother. Forceps delivery can be performed, however, the selection of instrument is dependent on the experience of the operator.

There are three generally accepted indications to use a ventouse to aid delivery:

- prolonged pushing in the second stage of labour or maternal exhaustion
- fetal hypoxia in the second stage of labour, generally indicated by changes in the fetal heart rate
- maternal illness where 'bearing down' or pushing efforts would be risky (e.g. cardiac conditions, raised blood pressure).

Answer 144 (F) Low forceps

To cut short the second stage of labour instrumental delivery is needed. As vertex is at plus two station with occipito posterior position, low forceps is the most appropriate instrument. Failure rate of instrumental delivery in OP position is less likely if conducted by forceps rather than ventouse.

Maternal exhaustion is one of the indications for instrumental delivery.

Classification for operative vaginal delivery (adapted from ACOG 2000):

Outlet forceps: When the fetal scalp is visible without separating the labia and fetal skull has reached the pelvic floor. Sagittal suture is in the antero-posterior diameter or right or left occiputo anterior or posterior position (rotation does not exceed 45 degrees).

Low forceps: Leading point of the skull (not caput) is at station plus 2 cm or more and not on the pelvic floor.

Two subdivisions:
(a) rotation of 45 degrees or less
(b) rotation more than 45 degrees.

Mid forceps: Fetal head is 1/5 palpable per abdomen and leading point of the skull is above station plus 2 cm but below the ischial spines.

Two subdivisions:
(a) rotation of 45 degrees or less
(b) rotation more than 45 degrees.

High forceps: Not included in classification.

Answer 145 (L) Emergency caeserean section

Instrumental delivery is contraindicated as she has herpes simplex infection. Fetal scalp sampling should also to be avoided.

Options for questions 146 – 148

A	First degree	F	Sixth degree
B	Second degree	G	Fourth degree
C	Seventh degree	H	Third degree 3c
D	Third degree 3a	I	Fifth degree
E	Third degree 3b	J	Buttonhole tear

Instruction: For each question posed below, choose the single **most appropriate classification for perineal tear** from the A–J list above. The given option may be used once, more than once or not at all.

Question 146	A 26 year old primigravida is in labour and has a spontaneous vaginal delivery of a 3.6kg male baby. She had a quick delivery and episiotomy was not performed. The midwife calls for help as she notices that the perineum is torn after delivery. On examination, it is found that the anal mucosa and internal anal sphincter are intact while 75% of the external anal sphincter is torn.
Answer 146	
Question 147	A 30 year old diabetic woman has just delivered a 4kg female baby with the help of forceps. Episiotomy was done after the application of forceps. After completion of delivery, extension of episiotomy was noticed. She was taken to theatre. On examination, it is found that the anal mucosa is torn along with the internal anal sphincter and the external anal sphincter.
Answer 147	
Question 148	A primigravida has delivered at 41 weeks of gestation. It was an occipito posterior delivery. Birth weight was 3.5kg. Perineal tear was noticed. Both external and internal anal sphincter are torn while the anal mucosa is intact.
Answer 148	

Answers and explanations

Answer 146 (E) Third degree tear 3b: More than 50% of EAS thickness torn

Most women during childbirth have some degree of perineal tear (85%) and in some the tear may be more extensive (1–9%).

Answer 147 (G) Fourth degree

Injury to the perineum involving the anal sphincter complex (EAS and IAS) and anal epithelium is defined as fourth degree.

Answer 148 (H) Third degree 3c: Both EAS and IAS torn

Classification of perineal tear

First degree: Injury to perineal skin only.

Second degree: Injury to perineum involving perineal muscles but not involving the anal sphincter.

Third degree: Injury to perineum involving the anal sphincter complex:

3a: Less than 50% of EAS thickness torn.
3b: More than 50% of EAS thickness torn.
3c: Both EAS and IAS torn.

Fourth degree: Injury to perineum involves the anal sphincter complex (EAS and IAS) and anal epithelium.

Risk factors for perineal tear are:

1. Nulliparity
2. Asian or Indian sub-continent ethnicity
3. Woman with genital mutilation
4. Large baby in relation to maternal size (> 4kg)
5. Previous history of anal sphincter injury or perineal trauma requiring repair
7. Precipitate or faster than expected second stage
8. Instrumental birth
9. Active second stage longer than 1 hour
10. Midline episiotomy or an inadequately angled mediolateral episiotomy.

Options for questions 149 – 150

A	Caesarean delivery	F	Laxatives
B	Vaginal delivery	G	Prophylactic episiotomy
C	Broad-spectrum antibiotics	H	Endo-anal ultrasonography
D	Referral to a specialist colorectal surgeon	I	Physiotherapy and pelvic-floor exercises for 6–12 weeks
E	Reassurance	J	Anorectal manometry

Instruction: For each question posed below, choose the single most appropriate answer from the A–J list above. The given option may be used once, more than once or not at all.

Question 149	A 26 year old woman has visited her GP as she is experiencing pain and incontinence of flatus 10 weeks after delivery. She had a normal vaginal delivery but had an extension of episiotomy. It was third degree perineal tear, which was repaired by registrar.
Answer 149	
Question 150	A 30 year old primigravida had forceps delivery. She delivered a 3.75kg female baby. She had third degree tear. She is being discharged from hospital after successful repair. She has been prescribed antibiotics and laxatives.
Answer 150	

Answers and explanations

Answer 149 (D) Referral to a specialist colorectal surgeon

She should be referred to specialist colorectal surgeon for assessment. Endoanal USG and manometry is recommended, which can provide information about the defect including its length, maximum thickness of the external anal sphincter and the quality of the internal sphincter ring. Manometry assesses tone and contractile function of the sphincter. Secondary sphincter repair might be necessary in a small number of women by a colorectal surgeon.

Answer 150 (I) Physiotherapy and pelvic-floor exercises for 6–12 weeks

Pelvic floor exercise rehabilitates the tone and strength of musculature of the pelvis.

Options for questions 151 – 154

A	MMR vaccine may be given with anti-D injection in same limbs and with same syringes	**H**	MMR vaccine may be given with anti-D injection in same limbs and with different syringes
B	MMR vaccine cannot be given with anti-D injection	**I**	MMR vaccine to be given 3 months after anti-D injection
C	MMR vaccine may be given with anti-D injection in different limbs and with different syringes	**J**	MMR vaccine to be given one month after anti-D injection
D	MMR vaccine to be given six weeks after anti-D injection	**K**	Pregnancy should be avoided for one month
E	Pregnancy should be avoided for three months	**L**	Pregnancy should be avoided for six months
F	Stop breastfeeding for two days	**M**	Breastfeeding may be continued
G	Stop breastfeeding for two weeks	**N**	Stop breastfeeding for a week

Instruction: For each question posed below, choose the single most appropriate answer from the list above. The given option may be used once, more than once or not at all.

Question 151	A 23 year old primigravida has delivered normally a male baby of 3.5kg. Her blood group is B negative. Blood group of baby is B positive. During the antenatal period she was found to be rubella seronegative and was advised MMR vaccination postnatally.
Answer 151	
Question 152	A 34 year old primigravida delivered a 2.7kg female baby by LSCS. CS was done for breech presentation. Her blood group is A negative and blood group of the baby is A positive. She has been given anti-D injection. It is noticed just before discharge that she was seronegative for rubella and was advised MMR vaccination postnatally.
Answer 152	
Question 153	A 36 year old primigravida was found to be seronegative for rubella during the antenatal period. She received MMR vaccine postnatally. She is anxious to know whether she can continue with breastfeeding. The midwife has come to you for advice.
Answer 153	
Question 154	A 30 year old woman has come for pre-conception counselling. She was found to be seronegative for rubella and was advised vaccination. She wants to know how long she should avoid pregnancy for because of this.
Answer 154	

Answers and explanations

Answer 151 (C) MMR vaccine may be given with anti-D injection in different limbs and using different syringes

Answer 152 (I) MMR vaccine to be given 3 months after anti-D injection

MMR and anti-D may be given in the postpartum period and separate syringes and into different limbs should be used.

If not given simultaneously, MMR should be given 3 months after anti-D (Rh0) immunoglobulin as the efficacy of this vaccine may be reduced if it is administered during this period.

Answer 153 (M) Breastfeeding may be continued

Women should be advised that pregnancy should be avoided for 1 month after receiving MMR, but breastfeeding may continue.

Answer 154 (K) Women should be advised that pregnancy should be avoided for 1 month after receiving MMR

The percentage of rubella-susceptible pregnant women has increased over recent years. Therefore it would be prudent to ensure all rubella nonimmune women be vaccinated prior to discharge from the maternity ward.

Maternal rubella infection in the first 8–10 weeks of pregnancy results in fetal damage in up to 90% of infants. Multiple defects are common and collectively they are known as congenital rubella syndrome.

There is no evidence to suggest that administration of a rubella vaccine to a pregnant woman presents a risk for her fetus (although such a risk cannot be excluded on theoretical grounds). Therefore, women of a childbearing age should receive rubella vaccines (rubella, MR, or MMR vaccine) only if they state that they are not pregnant and only if they are counselled not to become pregnant for 1–3 months after vaccination. Women of a childbearing age who do not have documentation of rubella vaccination or serologic evidence of rubella immunity should be vaccinated with MMR, if they have no contraindications to the vaccine.

Options for questions 155 – 157

A	Continue to monitor and assess	G	Within six hours of birth
B	Within one hour	H	Within four hours
C	Within one hour of birth	I	Within half an hour
D	Within three hours of birth	J	Within two hours of birth
E	After four hours	K	Within two hours
F	Potentially serious situation, which needs appropriate action to be taken soon	L	Life-threatening or potential life-threatening situation, evaluate for pre-eclampsia

Instruction: For each question posed below, choose the single most appropriate answer from the list above. The given option may be used once, more than once or not at all.

Question 155	A 30 year old third gravida has just delivered. It was a normal vaginal delivery and pregnancy was uncomplicated throughout. The labour ward is very busy and the midwife wants to know the minimum duration before which one measurement of blood pressure should be documented.
Answer 155	
Question 156	A 34 year old second gravida has delivered a 3.5kg male baby. It was an instrumental delivery for maternal exhaustion. Blood pressure was 136/96 mmHg two hours after delivery. She is otherwise fine with no complaints. The midwife wants to know when to check her blood pressure again.
Answer 156	
Question 157	A 30 year old primigravida has delivered normally. Her blood pressure one hour after delivery was 140/90 mmHg. It was checked again after 2 hours and it was found to be 140/96 mmHg. She is complaining of headache and epigastric pain.
Answer 157	

Answers and explanations

Answer 155 (G) Within six hours of birth

A minimum of one blood pressure measurement should be carried out and documented within 6 hours of the birth. Eclampsia occurring more than 48 hours after delivery is known as late postpartum eclampsia. This was thought to be uncommon. However, recent evidence suggests that its incidence is increasing. In addition, the presentation of late postpartum pre-eclampsia/eclampsia may differ from that occurring during the antenatal period. This contributes to difficulty in diagnosing in an emergency department setting.

Answer 156 (H) Within four hours

If diastolic blood pressure is greater than 90 mmHg and there are no other signs and symptoms of pre-eclampsia, measurement of blood pressure should be repeated within 4 hours.

Answer 157 (L) Life-threatening or potential life-threatening situations, evaluate for pre-eclampsia

If diastolic blood pressure is greater than 90 mmHg and does not fall below 90 mmHg within 4 hours, evaluation for pre-eclampsia is recommended.

Status levels (NICE guidelines)

Status	Classification
Emergency	Life-threatening or potential life-threatening situation
Urgent	Potentially serious situation, which needs appropriate action
Non-urgent	Continue to monitor and assess

Options for questions 158 – 160

A	Respiratory physiotherapy should not be offered routinely	G	Respiratory physiotherapy can be offered
B	When they feel thirsty and hungry	H	It has to be decided by physiotherapist
C	After 24 hours	I	Not before 6 hours
D	After 12 hours	J	After 8 hours
E	24 hours after the last epidural 'top up' dose	K	As early as 4 hours after CS
F	12 hours after the last epidural 'top up' dose	L	6 hours after the last epidural 'top up' dose

Instruction: For each question posed below, choose the single most appropriate answer from the A–L list above. The given option may be used once, more than once or not at all.

Question 158	A 36 year old primigravida had a CS done for breech presentation. CS was uncomplicated and a live male baby of 3kg was delivered. She is enquiring when to eat and drink.
Answer 158	
Question 159	A 30 year old woman was induced at 37 weeks for IUGR. She had an epidural for pain relief. Emergency LSCS was done as CTG trace was pathological. When should her catheter be removed?
Answer 159	
Question 160	A third gravida was induced for postdate at 41 weeks. She was contracting 4 in 10. She had pethidine for gas relief. Suddenly the midwife noticed deceleration in fetal heart and vaginal examination showed cord prolapse. A category one LSCS was done under general anesthesia. A new midwife is enquiring about respiratory physiotherapy.
Answer 160	

Answers and explanations

Answer 158 (B) When they feel thirsty and hungry

After an uncomplicated CS a woman can eat and drink when they feel hungry or thirsty.

Answer 159 (F) 12 hours after the last epidural 'top up' dose

Once a woman is mobile, the urinary bladder catheter can be removed. If regional anaesthesia was given then it should be after the last epidural 'top up' dose.

Answer 160 (A) Respiratory physiotherapy should not be offered routinely

Routine respiratory physiotherapy has not been shown to improve respiratory outcomes.

(Reference – RCOG Green-top guidelines nos.8, 26, 31, 45, 50, 51, 53, 55. NICE guidelines CG13 2004, CG 62 2008, CG 70 2008, CG 55 2007, CG37 2006)